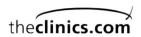

CRITICAL CARE NURSING CLINICS OF NORTH AMERICA

Genetics in Critical Care

GUEST EDITOR
Theresa A. Beery, PhD, RN, ACNP

CONSULTING EDITOR
Janet Foster, PhD, RN, CNS, CCRN

June 2008 • Volume 20 • Number 2

SAUNDERS

An Imprint of Elsevier, Inc.
PHILADELPHIA   LONDON   TORONTO   MONTREAL   SYDNEY   TOKYO

W.B. SAUNDERS COMPANY
A Division of Elsevier Inc.

Elsevier Inc., 1600 John F. Kennedy Blvd., Suite 1800, Philadelphia, PA 19103-2899.

http://www.theclinics.com

CRITICAL CARE NURSING CLINICS OF NORTH AMERICA   Volume 20, Number 2
June 2008   ISSN 0899-5885
Editor: Ali Gavenda   ISBN-13: 978-1-4160-5773-4
                                                                                  ISBN-10: 1-4160-5773-0

Reprints. For copies of 100 or more, of articles in this publication, please contact the Commercial Reprints Department, Elsevier Inc., 360 Park Avenue South, New York, New York 10010-1710. Tel. (212) 633-3813, Fax: (212) 462-1935, e-mail: reprints@elsevier.com.

The ideas and opinions expressed in *Critical Care Nursing Clinics of North America* do not necessarily reflect those of the Publisher. The Publisher does not assume any responsibility for any injury and/or damage to persons or property arising out of or related to any use of the material contained in this periodical. The reader is advised to check the appropriate medical literature and the product information currently provided by the manufacturer of each drug to be administered to verify the dosage, the method and duration of administration, or contraindications. It is the responsibility of the treating physician or other health care professional, relying on independent experience and knowledge of the patient, to determine drug dosages and the best treatment for the patient. Mention of any product in this issue should not be construed as endorsement by the contributors, editors, or the Publisher of the product or manufacturers' claims.

Critical Care Nursing Clinics of North America (ISSN 0899-5885) is published quarterly by Elsevier Inc., 360 Park Avenue South, New York, NY 10010-1710. Months of issue are March, June, September, and December. Business and Editorial Offices: 1600 John F. Kennedy Blvd., Suite 1800, Philadelphia, PA 19103-2899. Customer Service Office: 6277 Sea Harbor Drive, Orlando, FL 32887-4800. Periodicals postage paid at New York, NY and additional mailing offices. Subscription prices are $120.00 per year for US individuals, $212.00 per year for US institutions, $63.00 per year for US students and residents, $155.00 per year for Canadian individuals, $260.00 per year for Canadian institutions, $166.00 per year for international individuals, $260.00 per year for international institutions and $86.00 per year for Canadian and foreign students/residents. To receive student/resident rate, orders must be accompanied by name of affiliated institution, data of term, and the *signature* of program/residency coordinator on institution letterhead. Orders will be billed at individual rate until proof of status is received. Foreign air speed delivery is included in all *Clinics* subscription prices. All prices are subject to change without notice. **POSTMASTER:** Send address changes to *Critical Care Nursing Clinics of North America*, Elsevier Periodicals Customer Service, 6277 Sea Harbor Drive, Orlando, FL 32887-4800. **Customer Service: 1-800-654-2452 (US). From outside of the US, call 1-407-563-6020. Fax: 1-407-363-9661. E-mail: JournalsCustomerService-usa@elsevier.com.**

Critical Care Nursing Clinics of North America is covered in *International Nursing Index, Nursing Citation Index, Cumulative Index to Nursing and Allied Health Literature, and RNdex Top 100.*

Printed in the United States of America.

CONSULTING EDITOR

JANET FOSTER, PhD, RN, CNS, CCRN, Assistant Professor, College of Nursing, Texas Woman's University, Houston, Texas

GUEST EDITOR

THERESA A. BEERY, PhD, RN, ACNP, Professor, College of Nursing, University of Cincinnati, Cincinnati, Ohio

CONTRIBUTORS

SHEILA A. ALEXANDER, RN, PhD, Assistant Professor, Department of Acute and Tertiary Care, School of Nursing, University of Pittsburgh, Pittsburgh, Pennsylvania

MICHAEL BEACH, MSN, ACNP-BC, Instructor, Department of Acute and Tertiary Care, School of Nursing, University of Pittsburgh, Pittsburgh, Pennsylvania

THERESA A. BEERY, PhD, RN, ACNP, Professor, College of Nursing, University of Cincinnati, Cincinnati, Ohio

CHRISTOPHER FOWLER, PhD, RN, ACNP, Director, Transplant Clinical Operations, Transplant Services, Methodist Dallas Medical Center, Dallas; and Assistant Clinical Professor, School of Nursing, University of Texas at Arlington, Arlington, Texas

ROBERT B. HINTON Jr., MD, Assistant Professor of Pediatrics, Division of Cardiology, Cincinnati Children's Hospital Medical Center, Cincinnati, Ohio

CAROLE KENNER, DNS, RNC, FAAN, President, Council of International Neonatal Nurses (COINN), Edmond; and Dean and Professor, College of Nursing, University of Oklahoma, Oklahoma City, Oklahoma

JUDITH A. LEWIS, PhD, RNC, FAAN, Professor Emerita, School of Nursing, Virginia Commonwealth University, Richmond, Virginia

CINDY M. LITTLE, PhD, RNC, Senior Lecturer, Old Dominion University, Norfolk, Virginia

JANA L. PRESSLER, PhD, RN, Assistant Dean Research/Professor, College of Nursing, University of Oklahoma, Oklahoma City, Oklahoma

CYNTHIA A. PROWS, MSN, RN, FAAN, Clinical Nurse Specialist, Divisions of Patient Services and Human Genetics, Cincinnati Children's Hospital Medical Center, Cincinnati, Ohio

CHRIS WINKELMAN, RN, PhD, CCRN, ACNP, Assistant Professor, Frances Payne Bolton School of Nursing, Case Western Reserve University, Cleveland, Ohio

M. LINDA WORKMAN, PhD, RN, FAAN, Volunteer Faculty, College of Nursing, University of Cincinnati, Cincinnati, Ohio

VICKI L. ZEIGLER, PhD, RN, Assistant Professor, College of Nursing, Texas Woman's University, Denton, Texas

CONTENTS

Becoming comfortable with the onslaught of genetic information requires a familiarity with genetics terminology and basic molecular genetics. Caring for the genetic health of our patients requires an additional appreciation of genetic testing and screening issues and new areas of study with strange-sounding names, such as proteomics, nutrigenomics, and epigenetics. This article provides an overview of basic genetic principles and terminology with applications to critical care patients. It lays a foundation to support understanding of the other articles in this issue. An appreciation of genetics (the study of heredity) and genomics (the study of the interaction of genes within an organism) has an important place in the knowledge base of every critical care clinician.

Genetics has transformed the use of family history information and has led to the reemergence of the detailed genetic family history. It is critical that public and professional educational efforts to increase family history awareness and working knowledge are prioritized. Patient maintenance of the pedigree provides increased patient awareness and facilitates some of the limitations associated with conventional medical history ascertainment, ultimately improving health care and research. The increasing use of genetic screening promises to cultivate a paradigm shift in medical treatment emphasizing primary prevention and early intervention. Appreciation of the family history is necessary to make this important advance.

Improvements in the diagnosis and treatment of congenital heart disease have drastically reduced the morbidity and mortality associated with such defects. Knowledge regarding the genetic contributions to congenital heart disease is considered to be in its infancy; however, the field of cardiovascular genetics in humans is moving at a rapid pace. This article discusses what is currently known about the genetic contribution to congenital heart disease, including structural defects and congenital cardiac arrhythmias. Genetic and chromosomal syndromes that involve the heart are reviewed along with genetic testing.

pharmacogenetics is complex, the components of patient teaching are not beyond that which nurses already provide about other laboratory, disease, and treatment-based information. It is reasonable to expect that as the science of pharmacogenetics and pharmacogenomics expands and discoveries are translated in clinical settings, the additional information from pharmacogenetic test results will help prescribers select or adjust medication doses to reduce the risk for adverse drug reactions and improve the chances of achieving therapeutic targets in a timely fashion.

FORTHCOMING ISSUES

RECENT ISSUES

ELSEVIER
SAUNDERS

Crit Care Nurs Clin N Am 20 (2008) ix–x

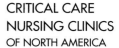

CRITICAL CARE
NURSING CLINICS
OF NORTH AMERICA

Preface

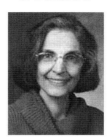

Theresa A. Beery, PhD, RN, ACNP
Guest Editor

The impact of genetics and genomics on understanding, preventing, and treating human diseases is undeniable. Clinical or research-based genetic testing is currently available for over 1,500 single gene diseases (www.genetests.org). Many of these are rare, not commonly seen outside of major medical centers or children's hospitals. The top causes of morality and morbidity in all ages (eg, coronary artery disease, osteoporosis, cancer, and hypertension) are complex (not single gene) diseases. These combine the effects of many genes working together or genes interacting with the environment. Nurses in all critical care settings see patients with chronic complex genetic diseases frequently.

Caring for the genetic health of our patients requires both an increased knowledge base and thinking about illness in new ways that include risk of present or future disease in family members as well as our patients. Nearly 50 nursing organizations have come together to publish *Essential Nursing Competencies and Curricula Guidelines for Genetics and Genomics* [1]. Genetics and genomics are both relevant and essential knowledge for all nurses.

This issue of *Critical Care Nursing Clinics of North America* provides articles covering foundational concepts and critical care applications of genetics and genomics. My own article begins the issue, presenting some basic tools, concepts, and terminology, to either refresh the reader's knowledge of genetics or bring up to date knowledge that has been out-paced by the rapid expansion of genetics and genomics following the Human Genome Project.

Dr. Hinton focuses his paper on the re-emergence of family history as a powerful tool in the critical care setting. He provides both basic content that is easily applied to practice and insights into the relevance of family history. Dr. Hinton offers the exemplar of family history in hypoplastic left heart syndrome based on his own clinical experience and laboratory research.

Several of the articles address genetics applications to specific sets of diseases. Dr. Zeigler reports current knowledge related to genetics and genomics and congenital heart disease. Drs. Workman and Winkelman discuss genetic and genomic influences in common pulmonary conditions, such as emphysema, bronchitis, and lung cancer. They also provide an overview of how genetic variants contribute to susceptibility and resistance. Dr. Fowler reviews the pathophysiology, diagnosis, and management of hereditary hemoschromatosis, which is the most common genetic disease in persons of European ancestry

0899-5885/08/$ - see front matter © 2008 Elsevier Inc. All rights reserved.
doi:10.1016/j.ccell.2008.02.001

[2]. An update of the genes involved in common neurologic diseases, such as multiple sclerosis, stroke, and intracerebral hemorrhage, is provided by Dr. Alexander and Mr. Beach. Dr. Winkelman provides an overview of the genes associated with infection and inflammation and also discusses the research methods used to identify them.

The use of genetics and genomics in personalizing pharmaceutic selection and dosing is increasing. Drs. Prows and Beery apply the science of pharmacogenetics to the treatment of atrial fibrillation. They include the timely example of genetic testing for warfarin response and the recent increase in availability of testing. Their article also reviews the *Essential Nursing Competencies and Curricula Guidelines for Genetics and Genomics* [1] and uses these to frame a discussion of the nurse's role in using pharmacogenetics.

The final article poses ethical questions relating to the use of newborn testing for genetic disorders. Dr. Kenner and colleagues consider whether it is ethical to perform a newborn genetic test when no treatment currently exists. They refer to genetic information nondiscrimination legislation and the importance of including a family history tool as a component of neonatal assessment.

As the guest editor, I would like to thank the authors for contributing their expertise and energy to provide an issue that will not only update readers, but will also challenge nurses to enhance the care they provide to their patients. Genetic advances are reported in the lay press and consumers of health care are becoming more knowledgeable about genetics and are asking more challenging questions. Genetics and genomics provide a relevant and dynamic tool to improve the quality of care for the critically ill.

Theresa A. Beery, PhD, RN, ACNP
Professor
College of Nursing
University of Cincinnati
PO Box 0038
Cincinnati, OH 45221-0038, USA

E-mail address: theresa.beery@uc.edu

References

[1] Consensus Panel of Genetic/Genomic Nursing Competencies: Essential Nursing Competencies and Curricula Guidelines for Genetics and Genomics. Silver Spring, MD: American Nurses Association; 2006.

[2] Tivall AS. Diagnosis and management of hemochromatosis. Hepatol 2001;33(5):1321–8.

Crit Care Nurs Clin N Am 20 (2008) 139–148

Genetics in Critical Care: A Toolbox

Theresa A. Beery, PhD, RN, ACNP

College of Nursing, University of Cincinnati, 3110 Vine Street, Cincinnati, OH 45221-0038, USA

Becoming comfortable with the onslaught of genetic information requires a familiarity with genetics terminology and basic molecular genetics. Caring for the genetic health of our patients requires an additional appreciation of genetic testing and screening issues and new areas of study with strange-sounding names, such as proteomics, nutrigenomics, and epigenetics. This article provides an overview of basic genetic principles and terminology with applications to critical care patients. It lays a foundation to support understanding of the other articles in this issue. An appreciation of genetics (the study of heredity) and genomics (the study of the interaction of genes within an organism) has an important place in the knowledge base of every critical care clinician.

Basic clinical genetics

Early discussions of genetics concentrated on single-gene disorders that were rare and affected mostly neonates. If you practiced in an adult critical care unit, genetics had little relevance to your daily work. Now the role of genetics/ genomics in common causes of adult morbidity and mortality is clear and genetic/genomics is making its presence known in every patient population. Genetics/genomics not only provides information predicting, diagnosing, or determining susceptibility to disease but also provides data on individualized responses to treatments and likely clinical course [1–3].

Diseases can be placed on a continuum according to the impact of genetics on disease expression from those that have a documented single-gene cause, such as Huntington disease, to those that

have more obscure genetic involvement, such as chicken pox (Fig. 1). Although infections do not, at first glance, seem to have genetic components, research is revealing many genetic reasons that some people become infected while others do not and why people's infections progress differently. Gene variants that indicate which people are more likely to develop sepsis and which people who have sepsis are more likely to progress to organ failure and death may one day be used to guide sepsis treatment [3–5].

Basic genetics jargon: you can't apply the principles if you don't speak the language

There has been a wealth of genetic information generated before and since the completion of the Human Genome Project [6]. To appreciate and understand it, a working knowledge of genetics concepts and terminology is needed. Fortunately, there are many excellent Web-based resources for becoming fluent in genetics at no cost. Access information for several Web sites is provided later in this article so you can expand your knowledge. This article provides a brief overview of what we are calling, "conversational genetics."

Chromosomes and genes

A chromosome is a threadlike package of DNA in the nucleus of a cell. Different kinds of organisms have different numbers of chromosomes. Humans have 23 pairs of chromosomes, 46 in all: 44 autosomes and 2 sex chromosomes (either XX or XY). Each parent contributes one chromosome of each pair, so children get one chromosome from their mothers and one chromosome from their fathers. A small bit of dad's DNA is added to each of mom's chromosomes and vice versa in a process called crossing over,

E-mail address: theresa.beery@uc.edu

doi:10.1016/j.ccell.2008.01.002

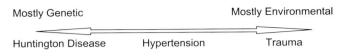

Mostly Genetic   Mostly Environmental

Huntington Disease   Hypertension   Trauma

Fig. 1. Continuum of genetic disease.

which occurs in one to two places on each chromosome and greatly increases the population's genetic diversity. Children inherit roughly 50% of their DNA from their mothers and 50% from their fathers. Siblings share about 50% of their DNA and grandparents and grandchildren share approximately 25% of their DNA [7].

Genes

A gene can be defined as a subunit of DNA, the physical unit of heredity that typically codes for proteins (Fig. 2). Humans have somewhere between 20,000 and 25,000 genes, which is not many more than the common roundworm (*Caenorhabditis elegans*) at about 19,000 and fewer than rice (*Oryza sativa*) at 30,000. Genes vary widely in size; for example, the gene that codes for somatostatin is only 1480 base pairs (bp), whereas dystrophin, the gene that is impaired in Duchenne muscular dystrophy, is more than 2,000,000 bp [8]. A gene this large offers many opportunities

for errors during replication or making messenger RNA.

DNA provides a blueprint or recipe book for directing the work of the cell. Most DNA is located in the cell's nucleus and most genetic diseases result from variations in nuclear DNA. A DNA molecule is a long string of chemical subunits called nucleotides (Fig. 3). Two strings of DNA are wrapped around each other and resemble a twisted ladder called the double helix. Phosphate and sugar molecules provide the scaffolding, but four nitrogen-containing bases connect the strings of nucleotides together using hydrogen bonds. The bases are adenine (A), guanine (G), cytosine (C), and thymine (T) and they connect in a specific way: A binds to T and G binds to C. When the two strands of DNA are bound together the G-C or A-T are referred to as base pairs (bps).

When cells divide the DNA unwinds at several locations, sometimes called bubbles, and free nucleotides bind to each of the original (parent) strands in the process of replication. This process results in production of exact copies of the original DNA for each of the new daughter cells [8,9]. Replication must be performed consistently and with great accuracy. Replication mistakes can result in long strings of unwanted repeated nucleotides

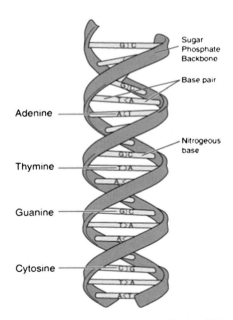

Fig. 2. Gene and chromosome. (*From* National Human Genome Research Institute. Talking glossary of genetics. Available at: www.genome.gov. Accessed October 17, 2007.)

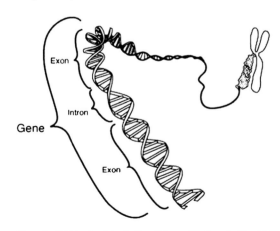

Fig. 3. DNA double helix. (*From* National Human Genome Research Institute. Talking glossary of genetics. Available at: www.genome.gov. Accessed October 17, 2007.)

that result in instability. Although repeats are common in the genome, expanded repeats (higher numbers of repeats) can be disease causing and are responsible for about 30 heritable disorders, such as Huntington disease and fragile X [10].

Sometimes a single base on the parent strand is replaced by a different base on the new strand. This single base change is called a substitution, and although it may seem insignificant, a single base substitution can result in disease. Sickle cell disease is caused by a substitution in the hemoglobin molecule [8]. Sometimes a base is added or deleted from the string of bases, which may result in production of a completely dysfunctional protein [8]. There are many ways that errors can be made in DNA replication or in the processes that follow. When genes are expressed they are turned on and they make a protein.

Making proteins

To make proteins, the DNA molecule unwinds again, and free nucleotides bind to their complementary bases forming a single-stranded molecule called messenger RNA (mRNA). This process is called transcription. While still in the nucleus, the noncoding regions (introns) are cut out of the transcribed sequence and the coding regions (exons) are joined together in a process called splicing. The ends are chemically capped, probably to provide stability to the molecule. The mRNA leaves the nucleus and travels out to the cytoplasm. The mRNA is used as a recipe to make protein the process of translation [9].

Translation is done according to the genetic code, which specifies the order of amino acids needed for that protein. For translation, each three-base unit of mRNA (called a codon) is "read" and the appropriate amino acid positioned in the correct order in the growing protein chain (Fig. 4). This process of placing all the right amino acids in the correct order (like beads on a string) continues until the protein strand is completely synthesized. Completion is signaled when a stop codon is read, indicating the end of the recipe for that protein. Some amino acids can be coded for by multiple codons, but there are three codons that indicate that the protein is complete and should be released from the ribosome. If there is a misspelling and a codon that should have coded for an amino acid is replaced by one of the STOP codons, the result is a shortened (truncated) protein, which will not function as expected. Some types of hereditary colon cancer can be caused by truncation mutations [9].

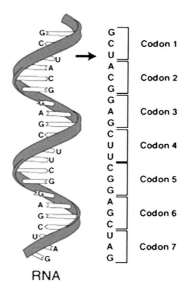

RNA

Ribonucleic acid

Fig. 4. mRNA and codons. (*From* National Human Genome Research Institute. Talking glossary of genetics. Available at: www.genome.gov. Accessed October 17, 2007.)

There are many additional small regulatory proteins that are involved by enhancing or silencing the processes of protein production. Proper transcription alone requires the involvement of about 50 different regulatory proteins. Sequence variations in some of these (eg, transcription factors) have also been associated with disease [11]. For example, mutations in the transcription factor *NKX 2.5* are associated with atrioventricular conduction block in some families [12].

Although all cells contain the entire genome, each cell makes different proteins as required. Protein production is based on physiologic need, which means that at any given time the variety and quantity of proteins produced will be different. We know that the beta cells of the pancreas make insulin and that they make more or less of it in response to blood glucose levels.

The collection of proteins produced at a given time and under specific conditions is called the proteome. Although the genome is stable over an organism's lifetime, the proteome changes constantly [9]. Once protein is made it must be folded properly to perform its expected function. The folding instructions are also coded in the DNA. Misfolded proteins are responsible for some forms of Alzheimer disease, cystic fibrosis, and mad cow disease (spongiform encephalopathy) [9].

Proteomics is the study of protein structures and functions and changes in protein production. There are more than 500,000 proteins coded for by our 20,000 to 25,000 genes, and slightly more than 40% have no known function as yet [7]. It is clear from looking at the number of genes in lower organisms that complexity is more closely related to protein product than the number of genes in the genome. We now know that genes can have multiple transcription start sites and that alternative splicing of mRNA can produce different proteins from the same gene sequence. Approximately 40% to 60% of genes produce multiple proteins, and some genes code for dozens of proteins. Proteins also can be altered after translation (posttranslational modification) by the removal or addition of chemical groups (such as phosphate, sugars, or fat to make phosphoproteins, glycoproteins, and lipoproteins) [7]. These mechanisms work together to make the thousands of different proteins needed by our cells.

Less than 5% of the 3 billion base pairs in the human genome actually code for protein (exons). The remainder of DNA includes sequences that provide regulation of replication and transcription and large portions of DNA about which we know little. These noncoding regions are of great interest to genetics researchers. They were originally believed to be unimportant, but there is increasing evidence of the role these variations play in disease and human variation [9]. Many of these variants are single nucleotide polymorphisms (SNPs).

Single nucleotide polymorphisms

SNPs are minute sequence variations in human DNA that are common and occur at a frequency of about 1 for every 1000 bp [13]. Common variations (polymorphisms) are typically not disease causing in themselves, but may function as modifiers of disease expression. Mutations are permanent changes in the DNA sequence. Generally DNA changes cause harm or have no effect, but occasionally a mutation can improve an organism's chance of surviving and the beneficial change is passed on to the organism's descendants [13]. There are some differences in how mutations and polymorphisms are defined. Some sources state that a mutation is a sequence change in an individual, whereas polymorphism refers to a change being evaluated on the population level [14].

Genetic diseases

Disorders with genetic components (some argue that all disorders have genetic components) can be classified as single-gene, chromosomal, mitochondrial or complex (multifactorial) disorders.

Single-gene disorders

Single-gene disorders can result from having one (dominant) or two (recessive) copies of a disease-causing mutation; the mutation may be located on one of the autosomes (autosomal) or on a sex chromosome (sex-linked). If a person carries two identical alleles (alternate form of a gene, one from the mother and one from the father) on each chromosome they are considered homozygous for that allele. If a person carries two different versions of a gene (eg, one normal [from either parent] and one mutant [from the other parent]) they are heterozygous. For example, hypercholesterolemia is an autosomal dominant single-gene disorder, caused by mutations in low-density lipoprotein (LDL) receptor gene or the apolipoprotein B gene (*APOB*) [14,15]. If a person has only one copy of the mutant gene, he or she has the genotype (the DNA sequence) for the disease. They may or may not have the phenotype (observable characteristics) of the disease. Some autosomal dominant diseases have incomplete penetrance, which means that not everyone who has the genotype necessarily has the phenotype [8]. See Box 1 for a summary of single-gene disorder transmission patterns.

Chromosomal disorders

Errors can happen when chromosomes are being allocated to germ cells (sperm and ova) and these are often profound because so many genes are carried by each chromosome. Sometimes chromosomes do not separate properly (nondisjunction) during the process of gamete production (meiosis). This nondisjunction can produce germ cells with two chromosomes from the mother rather than the expected single chromosome. When the egg is fertilized the embryo has three copies of that chromosome instead of two. This problem is called trisomy and depending on the chromosome involved it can be lethal. Most nurses are familiar with trisomy 21, or Down syndrome, because people who have this genetic variation can survive to birth and now into adulthood [8].

Trisomies of chromosomes 13 and 18 are usually lethal neonatally. Embryos with other trisomies typically do not survive to term [8]. The only monosomy that is viable is monosomy X or Turner syndrome. Girls who have Turner

Box 1. Modes of single-gene inheritance

Autosomal recessive inheritance
The gene involved is located on an autosomal chromosome and the genes on both chromosomes must be mutant to express the trait.

Autosomal dominant inheritance
The gene involved is located on an autosomal chromosome and only one gene must be mutant for expression of the trait.

X-linked recessive inheritance
The gene is located on the X chromosome and the genes on both chromosomes must be mutant to express the trait in females.
Because virtually all males only have one X chromosome, if that chromosome carriers a mutant form of the gene the trait is expressed.

X-linked dominant inheritance
The gene is located on the X chromosome and only one mutant gene is required for expression of the trait in females.
Because virtually all males only have one X chromosome, if that chromosome carriers a mutant form of the gene the trait is expressed. Often males are more severely affected, or they die prenatally.

Mitochondrial inheritance
The gene is located on the mitochondrial "chromosome."
There is maternal transmission.

syndrome have a characteristic appearance, including short stature, webbed neck, and shieldlike chest. Boys who are born with more than one X (most commonly XXY) have Klinefelter syndrome. Many boys who have Klinefelter syndrome do not realize that anything is wrong and are diagnosed in fertility clinics because they are unable to produce viable gametes [8].

Mitochondrial disorders

Some genetic diseases are caused by problems in mitochondrial DNA or the genes needed for cellular energy production by the mitochondria. These rare problems usually affect organs and tissues with high energy requirements and are frequently myoencephalopathies (muscle and brain problems) [8]. Because the mitochondria are located in the cytoplasm and virtually all cytoplasm comes from the egg rather than the sperm, mitochondrial inheritance is maternal. Even though males and females can be affected with mitochondrial disease, family histories show a pattern of transmission only through the mothers.

Complex disease

Most of the leading causes of morbidity and mortality (eg, cancer, coronary artery disease, diabetes mellitus type 2) are complex or multifactorial in origin. In these disorders small effects from many genes or combinations of genes and environment cause disease. In 2007 the American Heart Association issued a scientific statement on the relevance of genetics/genomics for prevention and treatment of cardiovascular (CV) disease [14]. The authors acknowledged that although some single-gene traits, (eg, hypercholesterolemia) are important in our understanding of CV disease, complex or multifactorial traits play the largest part in the diseases we see most commonly [14].

Hypertension is complex disease, largely because blood pressure maintenance requires the interaction of multiple organ systems (eg, vascular, renal, endocrine, neural) using complicated pathways that involve many different proteins [14]. It is extremely difficult to identify all genetic and environmental contributions in diseases such as these, but this is a major focus of current genetic research. The genes coding for proteins of the renin-angiotensin-aldosterone system have been studied, as have genes coding for inflammatory cytokines, adrenergic receptors, and endothelin. Results have been varied, indicating that susceptibility to hypertension is likely the result of an interaction among many gene variants and the environment (including personal environmental factors, such as obesity, sedentary lifestyle, and high-sodium diet) [16].

Delirium remains a significant problem in critical care. A recent study found an apolipoprotein E4 polymorphism that predisposes critically ill patients to longer episodes of delirium [17]. A review of studies looking at genetic predictors of delirium tremens found that although it is not a single-gene trait, a genetic link is certainly possible [18]. Further studies will provide evidence of whether genetic identification of at-risk patients can improve outcomes.

Genetic testing

There are currently clinical genetic tests for 1180 diseases available from Clinical Laboratory Improvement Amendments (CLIA)-certified laboratories. Clinical tests can be used for diagnosis, risk reduction, and treatment. Tests for an additional 283 diseases are available through participation in research studies; research results may not be provided to the patient and they are not to be used to direct patient care [19]. The numbers of both types of tests are growing rapidly as more gene variants causing or associated with disease are discovered.

The phrase "genetic testing" can be applied to diagnostic testing, predictive testing, carrier testing, prenatal testing, preimplantation testing, and newborn screening. DNA, RNA, certain metabolites, or chromosomes can be tested. Diagnostic testing is used to confirm the presence of a disease. For example, a child who has a borderline phenotype for long QT syndrome may be tested to see if she carries a variant in the genes that cause long QT [19].

Predictive genetic tests are given to asymptomatic people at risk for a given disease. Predictive tests are considered presymptomatic if a positive test means the patient will eventually get the disease. The test for Huntington disease is an example of a presymptomatic test. Predictive tests are predispositional if a positive result indicates that there is an increased risk for developing the genetic disease. The test for mutations in BRCA1/2 is predispositional, and if positive it denotes increased susceptibility to heritable breast cancer. Lifetime cumulative risk for developing breast cancer when one has a BRCA1 or BRCA2 mutation is approximately 86%. Lifetime risk for developing ovarian cancer in women who have BRCA1 mutations is variable but has been estimated at about 63% by age 70. Ovarian cancer risk in the presence of BRCA2 mutations is much lower, estimated at only 27% by age 70 [19].

Carrier testing is done for people (usually asymptomatic) who are at risk for passing on an autosomal recessive or X-linked recessive disease to their offspring. Usually there is an affected person in their family or the person requesting testing is of an ethnic group that is known to have a high incidence of carriers [19]. For example, about 1 in 30 people of Ashkenazi Jewish background is heterozygous for the gene mutation that causes the disorder of metabolism called Tay-Sachs. Because of a well-organized education and screening effort in the United States and Canada, births of children who have Tay-Sachs decreased by 90% from 1970 to the 1990s [8].

There are several genetic tests associated with pregnancy. Prenatal screening is provided during a pregnancy to assess the genetic risk of the fetus. Tests can include amniocentesis or chorionic villus sampling, both of which carry some risk to the fetus. Newborn screenings are also considered genetic tests. Although they are performed routinely at birth, the particular tests done differ among the states. All states require tests for phenylketonuria, galactosemia, and congenital hypothyroidism [20]. If parents do not want their child tested they must refuse the tests in writing. These are screening tests and if they are positive more definitive diagnostic tests must be completed to determine whether the infant actually has the disorder [19]. When there is a high likelihood of having a child who has a genetic disease (eg, both parents are carriers of gene mutations that can cause cystic fibrosis) some couples are choosing to have preimplantation genetic diagnosis. In this procedure, in vitro fertilization is done and the embryos are tested to find those free of the genetic condition of concern. Although it is expensive and somewhat controversial, this procedure provides an alternative to prenatal genetic testing and the decision about whether or not to terminate a pregnancy [19].

Direct-to-consumer marketing of genetic tests is becoming of concern with the increased prominence of the Internet. Supporters believe that marketing directly to consumers increases access and patient autonomy. Those opposed point out that consumers may choose to have genetic tests done without understanding the implications of the results or having support from genetics professionals who can provide counseling. The American Society of Human Genetics has issued a statement on direct-to-consumer genetic testing addressing concerns related to the context and quality of testing, unsubstantiated claims, and the need for consumers to make informed choices [21].

Expanding the evidence of genetic contributions to disease

Genetic tests are diverse and vary with the goal of the testing. Some testing that was originally developed for research is now being used for diagnostic and predictive testing. For example, polymerase chain reaction (PCR) is a laboratory-based method for amplifying small quantities of DNA and making it possible to sequence the nucleotides or identify sequence variations. The amplification process takes place within only a few hours. One hospital reduced the transmission rate of methicillin-resistant staphylococcus aureus (MRSA) on a critical care unit by using PCR to amplify the bacterial DNA rather than waiting for culture-based results to identify MRSA-infected patients. The comparatively fast process of PCR has decreased time to definitive treatment for a vulnerable patient population [22]. We are including a brief description of common genetic research methods used to uncover genetic contributions to disease because they are often discussed in the research and practice literature.

Genome-wide association studies

Genome-wide association studies (GWAS) are population-based studies typically involving 1000 cases and 1000 controls. They seek to identify a region of the genome associated with disease by finding SNPs (or other markers with a known location in the genome) that are more common in people with a disease than in those without it. According to the National Institutes of Health "GWAS are...defined as [studies] of genetic variation across the entire human genome that [are] designed to identify genetic associations with observable traits (such as blood pressure or weight), or the presence or absence of a disease or condition" [23]. The term association is also used when a sequence variant has been found in patients who have a given disease, but disease causation has not been established.

Linkage studies

Linkage studies typically use data from families of people affected with a given disorder. A large nuclear family with several affected and unaffected members can also be informative when using linkage analysis. In these studies, the goal is to identify a small region of the genome where affected family members share a variation not shared by unaffected family members. Linkage analysis has been used to find chromosomal regions that are linked to diabetic neuropathy in various populations [24,25].

Candidate gene studies

Once a likely region of the genome has been identified by linkage analysis or other means, the genes in that region can be evaluated to determine if it seems biologically plausible that mutations in any of these could cause the disease of interest. For example, if family members who have long QT syndrome share a sequence variation in chromosome 11 around the location of the potassium channel gene KCNQ1, that gene then becomes a positional candidate. Once it is established that a properly functioning potassium channel coded for by KCNQ1 makes an important contribution to effective repolarization of the cardiac action potential the gene also becomes a biologic candidate. That gene would then be a good candidate for further laboratory evaluation [26].

Microarrays

A microarray uses fluorescent probes and a high-density matrix of nucleic acids, protein, or tissue to study the interactions of many genes at the same time and gene expression in various tissues. Slides are read by a scanning microscope that identifies differences in the fluorescent signal. Microarrays can be used to determine which genes are expressed in a given tissue at a particular time (eg, a study identifying genes expressed in the atrium of people who have atrial fibrillation used microarrays) [13,27]. In addition, the multi-pathogen identification microarray detects 18 different pathogenic viruses and makes it possible to screen for all these organisms simultaneously [28].

Bioinformatics

Bioinformatics describes the use of computer-based systems to store, organize, analyze, and interpret biologic data. Given the volume of data generated by genetic/genomic studies, bioinformatics has become essential. Some genetics research is done entirely using computer databases and the extensive resources cataloged through bioinformatics tools. This type of research is called "in silico" because it is done entirely on a computer. A recent article used computer modeling to determine if two mutations in a sodium channel gene (*SCN5A*) could cause the electrocardiogram changes seen in long QT or Brugada syndromes [23,29].

New and unusual applications of genetics have evolved and these too may have a direct impact on the way we practice.

Nutrigenomics

Nutrigenomics describes the impact of diet on the ways in which genes are expressed. Nutrigenetics refers to the impact of one's genetic makeup on physiologic response to food [30,31]. Although this is a relatively new field, it has been suggested that vitamin and mineral supplementation could have a positive impact on heritable problems with DNA repair in diseases such as cancer and mitochondrial diseases [32]. Having an above-average intake of several micronutrients, including calcium, vitamin E, retinal, folate, vitamin B12, and nicotinic acid, reduces genome damage and supports DNA repair mechanisms. During the lifetime of an organism the genome is exposed to many environmental factors that cause DNA damage. These include ultraviolet radiation, ionizing radiation, and chemical carcinogens. Micronutrient deficiency is a recent addition to this list [30,31]. Efforts are being made to identify foods and dietary patterns that prevent DNA damage over time [30,31]. Although nutritional support has always been a valued nursing intervention in critical care, maintaining an abundant supply of micronutrients may be more important than we had imagined.

Epigenetics

Despite all that is known about the human genome there are still discrepancies in what we see clinically and what we see at the genotype level. Identical twins do not always get the same diseases and not all people who have mutations that cause long QT syndrome have the disease. These and other questions have led scientists to uncover additional layers of complexity in how we make the transition from genotype to phenotype. The process of epigenetics describes changes in gene expression and other genome functions that are heritable and modifiable but do not change the DNA sequence itself [33,34]. Epigenetic changes are attributable to processes, including the addition of chemical groups (methylation) to the DNA, modifications of the proteins (histones) the double helix winds around, and alterations in chromatin (the complex of DNA and protein that forms chromosomes).

Although the process of methylation has an important role in normal control of gene expression, epigenetic changes have also been linked to human diseases, such as cancer, cardiovascular and pulmonary diseases, and autoimmune and behavioral problems. Environmental factors, such as exposure to viruses, heavy metals, hormones, radioactivity, and tobacco smoke, have all been proposed as possible triggers for epigenetic change. Because epigenetic factors seem to be changeable, they have become an important target for innovative treatment of some cancers. Chemotherapeutic agents that function as DNA

Box 2. Web-based resources supporting genetics

Dolan Learning Center: http://www.dnalc.org/home.html. Provided by Cold Spring Harbor Laboratory, the Dolan Learning Center offers are variety of resources in support of genetics education.

Genetics and Your Practice: http://www.marchofdimes.com/gyponline/index.bm2. Sponsored by the March of Dimes this Web site provides information about genetic testing, collecting family and social history, and genetics referrals.

Genetics Home Reference http://ghr.nlm.nih.gov/. From the National Library of Medicine, this site provides a wealth of information for clinicians and consumers.

Gene.tests.org: http://www.genetests.org. Funded by the National Institutes of Health and maintained by the University of Washington, this Web site provides reviews of genetic diseases and locations of clinical and research genetic testing. Provides an excellent on-line genetics glossary.

National Human Genome Research Institute (NHGRI): http://www.genome.gov. Many resources for educational support, this site includes information of health policy and legal ethical issues related to genetics.

The Online Mendelian Inheritance in Man: http://www.ncbi.nlm.nih.gov/omim/. A catalog of human genes and genetic disorders developed by Dr. Victor A. McKusick and Johns Hopkins University. It provides textual and reference information, and links to the PubMed database and gene sequence information.

The University of Utah, Genetic Science Learning Center: http://gslc.genetics.utah.edu/. The GSLC offers a clear resource for basic genetics information, including animations.

methylation inhibitors are under investigation, with promising results [35].

Staying current

Staying current in genetics is a challenge with active genetics research projects producing results that augment or change our understanding of innate genetic processes and potential therapies. Textbooks are frequently outdated before they go to press. Web-based resources have become important sources of accurate and up-to-date genetic information. Animated tutorials can provide a review of basic genetic principles that are interactive and engage people who have varied learning styles. We have included an annotated listing of some of the most reliable, current, and usable Web sites for expanding and maintaining your genetic literacy (Box 2).

Summary

We have provided a set of tools to facilitate the clinician's ability to understand and use genetic concepts in the care of the critically ill patient, including concepts from molecular and clinical genetics, an overview of the classifications of genetic diseases, genetic terminology, and types of genetic testing used clinically and for research. We have also provided a few additional examples of applications of genetic research to critical care and introduced the topics of nutrigenomics and epigenetics. Staying current when the field of genetics/genomics is changing so rapidly continues to be a challenge for all critical care clinicians. This toolbox provides a useful resource.

Glossary

Allele: An alternate form of a gene at a particular location on a chromosome [13].
Alternative splicing: Producing different forms of mRNAs from the same gene by incorporating different exons, or coding regions; this process results in more than one protein being produced from a single gene sequence [7].
Chromosome: A connected collection of genes and other DNA that resides in the nucleus of a cell. A parent provides one of each chromosome to an offspring so that 50% of genetic material comes from the mother and 50% comes from the father [13].
Compound heterozygous: Having two different copies of a gene variant, neither of them wild type [8].

Epigenetics: Heritable and modifiable processes that affect activity of the genes but do not alter the DNA sequence [34].
Gene: The physical unit of heredity. Genes are segments of DNA and most code for proteins.
Genotype: The genetic constitution [8].
Genome: The entire collection of genes within an organism [13].
Heterozygous: Having two different copies of a gene, one wild type and one a variant [8].
Homozygous: Having two identical copies of a gene, either both wild type or both the same gene variant [8].
Locus: The position of a gene on a chromosome [7].
Mutation: An alteration in DNA structure that is permanent [13].
Nutrigenomics: The impact of diet on the ways in which genes are expressed [31].
Phenotype: Observable characteristics of an organism, which result from genes and environment [8].
Posttranslational modification: Changes, such as the addition or removal of chemical groups, made to a protein after translation [8].
Proteome: The protein expression within an organism at a particular point in time. Some scientists use this term to mean the complete set of proteins within a cell [7].
Single nucleotide polymorphisms (SNPs): Common single base variations in DNA sequence [13].
Splicing: The removal of noncoding regions (introns) from the transcribed sequence and the joining together of protein coding regions (exons) [7].
Transcription: The process by which DNA codes for messenger RNA [7].
Translation: The process by which mRNA codes for protein [7].
Wild type allele: The form of a gene that is most common in nature (the nonmutant form); often referred to as the "normal" form [7].

References

[1] Roden DM. Cardiovascular pharmacogenomics. Circulation 2003;108(25):3071–4.
[2] Weinshilboum R, Wang L. Pharmacogenomics: bench to bedside. Nat Rev Drug Discov 2004;3(9):739–48.
[3] Pinsky MR. Genetics of individualizing patient care. Crit Care Med 2007;35(1):287–90.
[4] Tabrizi AR, Zehnbauer BA, Freeman BD, et al. Genetic markers in sepsis. J Am Coll Surg 2001;192(1):106–17 [quiz: 145–6].

[5] Villar J, Maca-Meyer N, Perez-Mendez L, et al. Bench-to-bedside review: understanding genetic predisposition to sepsis. Crit Care 2004;8(3):180–9.

[6] NHGRI. Human genome project. Available at: http://www.genome.gov/10001772; 2007. Accessed August 24, 2007.

[7] Klug WS, Cummings MR, Spencer CA. Concepts of genetics. 8th edition. Upper Saddle River (NJ): Pearson - Prentice Hall; 2006.

[8] Jorde LB, Carey JC, Bamshad MJ, et al. Medical genetics. 3rd edition. St. Louis (MO): Mosby, Inc.; 2006.

[9] Cummings MR. Human heredity. 7th edition. Belmont (CA): Thomson Learning; 2006.

[10] Mirkin SM. Expandable DNA repeats and human disease. Nature 2007;447(7147):932–40.

[11] Clark KL, Yutzey KE, Benson DW. Transcription factors and congenital heart defects. Annu Rev Physiol 2006;68:97–121.

[12] Schott JJ, Benson DW, Basson CT, et al. Congenital heart disease caused by mutations in the transcription factor NKX2-5. Science 1998;281(5373):108–11.

[13] NHGRI. Talking glossary of genetic terms. Available at: http://genome.gov/10002096; 2007. Accessed August 15, 2007.

[14] Arnett DK, Baird AE, Barkley RA, et al. Relevance of genetics and genomics for prevention and treatment of cardiovascular disease: a scientific statement from the American Heart Association Council on Epidemiology and Prevention, the Stroke Council, and the Functional Genomics and Translational Biology Interdisciplinary Working Group. Circulation 2007;115(22):2878–901.

[15] Brown MS, Goldstein JL. A receptor-mediated pathway for cholesterol homeostasis. Science 1986; 232(4746):34–47.

[16] Puddu P, Puddu GM, Cravero E, et al. The genetic basis of essential hypertension. Acta Cardiol 2007; 62(3):281–93.

[17] Ely EW, Girard TD, Shintani AK, et al. Apolipoprotein E4 polymorphism as a genetic predisposition to delirium in critically ill patients. Crit Care Med 2007;35(1):112–7.

[18] van Munster BC, Korevaar JC, de Rooij SE, et al. Genetic polymorphisms related to delirium tremens: a systematic review. Alcohol Clin Exp Res 2007; 31(2):177–84.

[19] GeneTests. About genetic services. 3-19-04; Available at: http://www.genetest.org; 2007. Accessed October 17, 2007.

[20] NNSGRC. National newborn screening status report. 10-17-07; Available at: http://genes-r-us.uthscsa.edu/nbsdisorders.pdf; 2007. Accessed October 17, 2007.

[21] ASHG. ASHG statement on direct-to-consumer genetic testing in the United States. Am J Hum Genet 2007;81:635–7.

[22] Cunningham R, Jenks P, Northwood J, et al. Effect on MRSA transmission of rapid PCR testing of patients admitted to critical care. J Hosp Infect 2007;65(1):24–8.

[23] DHHS. Genome-wide association studies. Available at: http://grants.nih.gov/grants/gwas/index.htm; 2007. Accessed August 25, 2007.

[24] Krolewski AS, Poznik GD, Placha G, et al. A genome-wide linkage scan for genes controlling variation in urinary albumin excretion in type II diabetes. Kidney Int 2006;69(1):129–36.

[25] Ng DP, Krolewski AS. Molecular genetic approaches for studying the etiology of diabetic nephropathy. Curr Mol Med 2005;5(5):509–25.

[26] Beery TA, Dyment M, Shooner K, et al. A candidate locus approach identifies a long QT syndrome gene mutation. Biol Res Nurs 2003;5(2):97–104.

[27] Lamirault G, Gaborit N, Le Meur N, et al. Gene expression profile associated with chronic atrial fibrillation and underlying valvular heart disease in man. J Mol Cell Cardiol 2006;40(1):173–84.

[28] Wilson W, Strout C, DeSantis T, et al. Sequence-specific identification of 18 pathogenic microorganisms using microarray technology. Mol Cell Probes 2002;16(2):119–27.

[29] Vecchietti S, Grandi E, Severi S, et al. In silico assessment of Y1795C and Y1795H SCN5A mutations: implication for inherited arrhythmogenic syndromes. Am J Physiol Heart Circ Physiol 2007; 292(1):H56–65.

[30] Fenech M. Nutrition and genome health. Forum Nutr 2007;60:49–65.

[31] Fenech M. Genome health nutrigenomics and nutrigenetics—diagnosis and nutritional treatment of genome damage on an individual basis. Food Chem Toxicol 2008;46(4):1365–70.

[32] Ames BN. A role for supplements in optimizing health: the metabolic tune-up. Arch Biochem Biophys 2004;423(1):227–34.

[33] Gal-Yam EN, Saito Y, Egger G, et al. Cancer epigenetics: modifications, screening, and therapy. Annu Rev Med 2008;59:267–80.

[34] Ptak C, Petronis A. Epigenetics and complex disease: from etiology to new therapeutics. Annu Rev Pharmacol Toxicol 2007;48:257–76.

[35] Garcia-Manero G, Kantarjian HM, Sanchez-Gonzalez B, et al. Phase 1/2 study of the combination of 5-aza-2'-deoxycytidine with valproic acid in patients with leukemia. Blood 2006;108(10):3271–9.

ELSEVIER
SAUNDERS

Crit Care Nurs Clin N Am 20 (2008) 149–158

CRITICAL CARE
NURSING CLINICS
OF NORTH AMERICA

The Family History: Reemergence of an Established Tool

Robert B. Hinton Jr., MD

Division of Cardiology, MLC 2003, Cincinnati Children's Hospital Medical Center,
3333 Burnet Avenue, Cincinnati, OH 45229-3039, USA

There is a perception that the family history has played little if any role in the management of patients in an intensive care setting; the family history may be considered noncontributory in the context of caring for an acutely ill patient. The health care team is focused on stabilizing the patient and responding to acute, often life-threatening needs. To this end, patient evaluation is often restricted. The time-honored primary survey prioritizes assessment of "ABC" (airway, breathing, circulation) and has been expanded to include D for disability and E for exposure. A growing body of knowledge in human genetics and molecular medicine suggests that the family history is no longer limited to risk identification during obstetric prenatal counseling and ambulatory primary care, and may have direct applications in all areas of health care, including the intensive care unit. For example, consider the postoperative patient who has bleeding who has a positive family history of von Willebrand disease. Knowledge of the family history in this case would guide the diagnostic work-up and direct management in a timely manner. In light of the potential value of family history information and the expanding use of genetic information, it may be time to include F for family history in the primary survey.

A detailed family history provides the first genetic screen for an individual and contains substantial medical information; however, many patients are unaware of their own family histories and health care providers underuse it. As genetic testing becomes available and more commonly used, and the medical field embraces primary prevention and early intervention, the genetic family history will become increasingly important in clinical decision making, especially before overt disease manifestation. Many efforts are currently being directed toward increasing awareness of the value of the family history and identifying efficient ways to implement the use of family history information.

The purpose of this article is to define the genetic family history, describe the practical use of the pedigree in interpreting the family history, and describe how genetics is leading to the reemergence of family history use. An example describing ascertainment of the family history illustrates the value of a detailed family history. In addition to its role as an essential tool for the geneticist, family history has a central usefulness for all health care providers and renewed impact on clinical management in the emerging genetic era.

The family history

The origins of the family history

The origins of the medical family history ultimately trace to genealogy. Genealogy is the study of a person's identity as defined by ancestry and vital records. Typically, this includes an extended family tree defining biologic relationships and certificates documenting basic milestones in life, such as birth, marriage, and death. The death certificate often includes the cause of death and is essentially a piece of medical

This work was supported by a Trustee Award from the Children's Hospital Research Foundation (Cincinnati, Ohio) and a grant from the National Institutes of Health HL085122.

E-mail address: robert.hinton@cchmc.org

information. In addition, facts regarding education, occupation, and medical health are often compiled. Taken together, this collection of information defines an individual as part of a larger biologic system, namely the family, and the family tree identifies among other things the patterns of disease present in a particular family. Genealogy therefore defined many of the basic tenets of the medical family history.

The medical family history traces to antiquity. Hippocrates is generally credited with developing case histories, which included observations regarding the importance of family history in addition to clinical evaluation in the role of disease manifestation [1]. His emphasis on prognosis, at a time when treatment was limited, was largely informed by the observation that disease type and severity often seemed to run in families; this was the precursor to risk stratification. The modern medical family history is a record of illnesses and other pertinent health issues among family members [2]. Conventional, albeit underused, applications of the family history include confirming medical diagnoses, identifying family members at risk for various conditions, and calculating risk for developing a particular disease [3–5].

As more is learned about the genetic basis of disease, the family history has evolved into the first genetic screen. Since the experiments of Gregor Mendel [6], an Austrian priest, in the mid 1800s, our understanding of genetic information has been increasing exponentially. Mendel was interested in the theory of evolution and specifically how atypical traits developed in plants. His experiments recording the inheritance of traits in pea plants were reported in 1865; however, they were not appreciated for nearly 40 years until after his death when his paper "Experiments in Plant Hybridization" was translated into English and published in the *Journal of the Royal Horticultural Society* in 1901. This study stands as the basis of our understanding of heredity and heralded the study of modern human genetics. Taken together, genetic information promises to complement and advance the value of the family history.

Obtaining the family history

A medical family history can be abbreviated or detailed [2]. An abbreviated family history entails questioning the person of interest. This approach, however, is prone to misinformation and omission because it relies on the knowledge and memory of one person. Several screening tools have been

developed to obtain a cursory family history, such as SCREEN (Table 1) [7], which identifies general family history information and areas in need of more detailed information. This approach is a useful starting point in obtaining a detailed or complete family history. Ascertainment of medical history can be both open-ended and focused on a specific organ system. For example, common disease categories may be reviewed initially, including coronary artery disease, diabetes, hypertension, breast/ovarian cancer, colon cancer, mendelian conditions, and reproductive risk; subsequently the answers to these broad questions can direct the ascertainment of detailed organ-specific information.

A detailed family history refers to questioning multiple individuals within a family and requires specific demographic information (eg, age at disease onset) and documentation of disease and other pertinent health issues by medical record review. For example, when the initial review reveals a family history significant for coronary artery disease, problem-specific questions pertaining to the cardiovascular system may be pursued, including those listed in Box 1 [2,8,9]. This approach can be applied to all relevant organ systems in obtaining a detailed family history. This practice is time intensive and unfortunately generally reserved for clinical genetics and research purposes; however, it is easy to appreciate the clinical value of exhaustively collected, organized, and accessible family history information. The results of a detailed family history may warrant referral to a genetics service. The indications for referral are context specific and may include known genetic conditions, multiple family members with the same condition, and the presence of congenital

Table 1
Abbreviated family history: SCREEN for familial disease

SC	Some concern	Do you have any concern about diseases that run in the family?
R	Reproduction	Have there been complicated pregnancies, infertility, or birth defects?
E	Early disease/death	Has anyone in your family become sick or died at an early age?
E	Ethnicity	How would you describe your ethnicity?
N	Nongenetic	Are there risk factors that run in your family?

Box 1. Detailed family history: questions for cardiac disease

Information on family members

Is there a history of coronary artery disease, cardiomyopathy, arrhythmia, or congenital heart disease?

Is there a history of sudden death or childhood death? What age? (obtain reports)

Is there a history of pregnancy loss?

Is there a history of consanguinity?

Does anyone have a pacemaker?

Does anyone need to take antibiotics before medical/dental procedures?

Does anyone have facial dysmorphology? (genetic syndromes often associated with cardiac malformation)

Is there a history of neuromuscular disease? (Duchenne muscular dystrophy, Friedreich ataxia)

Is there a history of hearing loss? (LQTS)

Is there a history of unusual skin findings? (dyslipoproteinemias and connective tissue disorders)

Is there a history of unusually short or tall stature? (Marfan, Turner, and Noonan syndromes)

Is there a history of loose joints? (Marfan and Ehlers-Danlos syndromes)

Information on affected individuals

At what age was heart disease diagnosed?

Is the person living or deceased? (if deceased, obtain autopsy report)

Does this person have other medical problems?

Has surgery been performed? (obtain operative and pathology reports)

Have diagnostic studies been performed? (obtain reports)

What medications does the person take?

Is there a history of alcohol or tobacco use? How much?

---

malformations [10,11]. A detailed family history can help establish a diagnosis and initiate comprehensive care when needed.

Constructing the pedigree

A pedigree, also known as a family tree, is a graphic representation of a family history using symbols [2,12]. The pedigree is used for many clinical and research purposes, including making a diagnosis, establishing a pattern of inheritance, identifying family members at risk, calculating risk, deciding testing and surveillance strategies, and patient education [2,13–16]. Importantly, the pedigree facilitates a patient's understanding of disease by illustrating the central observations of a medical family history and promoting conversation that clarifies misconceptions about disease and heritability. The pedigree is the primary mode of communication in clinical genetics and human genetics research. Given the universal use of this tool, the National Society of Genetic Counselors formed a Pedigree Standardization Task Force and developed standard nomenclature for pedigrees [17]. As a result of this effort, there is a system of common symbols used to consistently communicate relationships and health status. Because the family history impacts all areas of medicine, it is important that all health care professionals have a working knowledge of pedigree structure.

A complete pedigree includes identification of the index case or proband (the person of interest) and detailed medical history as described above from at least three generations. The family is organized by generation, such that each generation is on a different line and designated by sequential Roman numerals from top to bottom and each individual is given an Arabic number reading from left to right (Fig. 1C). This numbering system facilitates analysis by allowing easy identification of individuals. Lines connect the symbols and establish relationships. An arrow identifies the index case. Squares designate males, circles designate females, and diamonds designate unknown gender or multiple individuals. Different parts of a symbol may be filled in to represent specific medical conditions, and a legend is provided for precise reporting. In addition to illnesses,

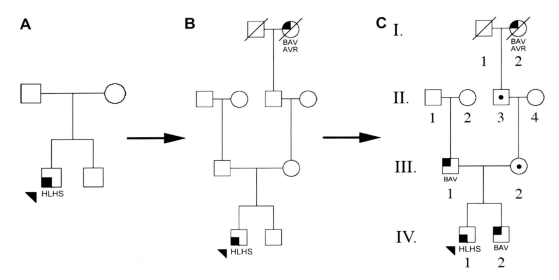

Fig. 1. The development of a detailed complete family history. After a new diagnosis of HLHS was established in an infant (IV-1, *arrowhead*), an abbreviated family history was noted to be noncontributory (*A*). On ascertainment of a detailed family history obtained from multiple family members (*B*), the family history was noted to be significant for BAV requiring AVR in a maternal great-grandmother (I-2). On screening echocardiography, two cases of subclinical BAV were discovered (III-1 and IV-2, (*C*) revealing a family enriched for cardiovascular malformation. Individuals II-3 and III-2 are obligate carriers (*dots*). Pedigree analysis is consistent with autosomal recessive inheritance with reduced penetrance. AVR, aortic valve replacement; BAV, bicuspid aortic valve; HLHS, hypoplastic left heart syndrome.

other significant health information can be recorded, including death, miscarriage, and twinning. A question mark indicates that medical information for a particular person is unknown or unavailable. It is important for clinical risk stratification and human genetics research to distinguish an individual who has an unknown status from an individual who has been evaluated and is known to be normal. Accurate and precise individual evaluation cannot be overemphasized. Because genetic information has become increasingly available, genetic data are often incorporated into the pedigree. A plus sign associated with a symbol indicates the presence of a particular genotype. A carefully constructed pedigree provides a succinct illustration of the family history and can be a powerful tool for patient education, genetic counseling, and research.

The family history is dynamic; medical information within families changes over time and needs to be revisited and updated. Some affected individuals may develop different or related conditions. In addition, many "healthy," "normal" individuals may be diagnosed with disease later in life consequently changing the overall record of disease within the family significantly. Accordingly, the pedigree needs to be updated regularly.

Information on unaffected individuals is equally important. Once the detailed family history is obtained, significant time needs to be invested to maintain the accuracy and value of the information [18]. As family history awareness improves and health care providers invest more time in obtaining detailed family histories, a potential challenge will be keeping the information up-to-date and relevant.

Barriers to using the family history

There are significant barriers to the optimal use of family history information, primarily a lack of awareness on the family's part and considerable time restrictions on the health care professional's part. Studies have shown that most people do not know their family history and do not appreciate its relevance in medical management, and consequently the potential impact of family history information is diminished [3,19–21]. Several reports have shown that patients often have poor recall regarding their own diagnoses and limited knowledge regarding illnesses present within their family. In addition, parents of pediatric patients who have chronic diseases often do not know the specific diagnoses of their children [22]. In an effort to increase family history awareness, tools have been developed and are available to the general public to generate and maintain a detailed family history. For example, the Health and Human Services Family History Initiative has designed a publicly available, Web-based program providing a means to generate and maintain a detailed family history (for this and other resources, see Table 2) [3]. Efforts to improve family history awareness and develop comprehensive family history tools are ongoing.

The time investment required for thorough review of the family history often precludes completion of a detailed family history. In the ambulatory primary care setting, Acheson and colleagues [20] found that family history was discussed in only one half of new patient visits and less than one quarter of return visits. Further, when family history was discussed it was allotted less than 3 minutes' time. Taken together, these findings suggest that family history is selectively performed, abbreviated in nature, and suboptimally maintained [22,23]. The authors point out that time constraints in most health care settings, including the clinic, make it difficult to complete an abbreviated family history, let alone a detailed or updated family history. In addition to significant practical limitations, many health care providers, including doctors, do not have formal training in genetics and are not comfortable with genetic counseling [19,24]. Nursing, however, has taken the lead in educating health care professionals to increase the hands-on use of genetic information [25]. One potential approach entails organizing family history information by sending patients a detailed questionnaire to be filled out before the encounter and providing resources at the time of the visit to develop and maintain their family history. Efforts to prioritize family history information will ultimately require overcoming major limitations in a creative way, potentially including increased patient involvement in record maintenance and increased resource allocation by health care administration.

Family history as patient empowerment

Public health initiatives have recommended using the medical family history as an educational tool and developing a comprehensive record that can be kept by the patient requiring only regular updating [4,24,26]. This practice would accomplish increased awareness of family history and compilation of important information that can be used in multiple medical contexts. For example, one may carry the family history and pedigree like an immunization record, so in the event of an emergency or new health concern that information is readily available. Public and professional education regarding the value of family history is needed. In addition, substantial resource allocation and organization is needed to effectively obtain, analyze, and maintain this sort of information. Increased family history awareness ultimately leads to increased medical awareness, and with increased understanding of health and disease there is probably improved adherence and better overall care.

How does genetics impact the family history?

Genotype–phenotype

An individual's genotype is a person's overall genetic constitution and may refer specifically to sequence variations that can cause or increase the susceptibility to disease. Informally, a person is genotype-positive if they have the sequence variation in question. An individual's phenotype is the observable characteristics of that individual, including, for example, eye color, serum cholesterol levels, or the presence of heart valve disease, such that the phenotype is the manifestation of the genotype. For instance, a person who has Williams-Beuren syndrome (MIM#194050) has a microdeletion on chromosome 7 resulting in the loss of function of several genes (genotype), which can manifest as dysmorphology, impaired cognition, and arteriopathy (phenotype). One genotype may result in different phenotypes and not all phenotypes are outwardly observable. Some phenotypic differences can only be appreciated after

Table 2
Resources for genetic family history ascertainment and awareness

Health and Human Services Family History Initiative	www.hhs.gov/familyhistory
Online Mendelian Inheritance of Man	www.ncbi.nlm.nih.gov/Omim
Centers for Disease Control	www.cdc.gov/genomics
March of Dimes	www.marchofdimes.com
National Coalition for Health Professional Education in Genetics	www.nchpeg.org
American Medical Association	www.ama-assn.org

laboratory analysis. There is increasing interest in genotype–phenotype relationships (ie, associations between specific genotypes and phenotypes that may be clinically informative). For example, in a patient who has Williams-Beuren syndrome, loss of function of the elastin gene within the microdeletion results in arteriopathy, whereas cognitive impairment has been attributed to loss of function of the LIMK1 gene. The ability to stratify specific phenotypes with specific genotypes informs our understanding of the mechanisms underlying disease and has the potential to direct medical care.

Heritability

Traits or illnesses within a family are often referred to interchangeably as familial or heritable; however, heritability has a more specific meaning. Traits are familial if members of the same family share them for any reason; traits are only heritable if the similarity arises specifically because of shared genotypes. Heritability is the proportion of phenotypic variation attributable to genetic effects. Heritability of human traits, including disease states, is estimated using careful phenotype data and complex statistical methods [27]. A high heritability suggests that major genetic effects cause a particular trait. A high heritability therefore predicts that genetic discovery studies (eg, linkage analysis and genome-wide association studies) should be able to identify disease loci and ultimately disease-causing gene mutations.

Pedigree analysis and human genetics research of heritable diseases can be confounded by several phenomena. Confounding factors include genetic heterogeneity, variable expressivity, and reduced penetrance. Genetic heterogeneity is present when different genotypes result in the same phenotype. Variable expressivity is present when the same genotype results in different phenotypes. Reduced penetrance is present when a specific genotype results in a phenotype only a proportion of the time (ie, there are individuals who have the genotype in question but do not manifest the phenotype). These phenomena are common and have been shown to be present in varying degrees in many diseases, including pediatric heart disease [28,29].

DNA sequence variation

A sequence variation may be a gene mutation or a polymorphism. In general, a mutation is a variation in DNA that leads to altered gene function. There are many types of mutations, including single base substitutions, insertions, and deletions. Mutations can be deleterious and result in disease or they can be neutral or beneficial. Polymorphisms are common sequence variations that are generally not believed to cause pathology directly. Classic mendelian diseases, such as inborn errors of metabolism, tend to be rare and are caused by gene mutations, whereas complex diseases (those caused by a combination of genetic and environmental factors), such as coronary artery disease or type 2 diabetes, tend to be common and associated with polymorphisms. For example, single nucleotide polymorphisms (SNPs) have been associated with an increased susceptibility or predisposition to disease. Although family history has been established as an independent risk factor for many common complex diseases, including coronary artery disease, hyperlipidemia, and type 2 diabetes [4,13,14,23,30,31], there is an increasing appreciation that polymorphisms may also identify disease susceptibility complementing the family history. Identification of a genotype in the presence or absence of a positive family history before the manifestation of disease may have significant implications. For example, screening strategies, treatment, and counseling may all be modified as a result of genotype knowledge. It remains unclear whether or to what extent the identification of sequence variations will provide an incremental benefit in risk stratification over family history information or will identify clinically relevant genotype–phenotype relationships.

Genetic screening for breast cancer: an example

Screening for mutations or polymorphisms that are associated with disease risk is now possible and can be performed in those considered at increased risk by family history. Because these markers can be identified before the development of disease, they may potentially lead to medical intervention before disease onset to delay or abrogate the manifestation of disease. Recently, a family was reported that illustrated the potential actions that can be taken by an individual who carries a gene mutation associated with disease but does not presently manifest any evidence of disease [32]. A 33-year-old woman who had a strong family history of breast and ovarian cancer decided to undergo screening and learned she carried a mutation in the BRCA1 gene. She was confronted with difficult and controversial options, including increased medical surveillance and preemptive removal of her breasts and ovaries. She decided to proceed with prophylactic mastectomy, deferring removal of her ovaries until after she has had children. The ability to make a diagnosis based on genetics before the onset of disease has the potential to shift the paradigm of medical treatment to primary prevention and early intervention.

Genetic screening for sudden cardiac death: an example

Hypertrophic cardiomyopathy and long QT syndrome are common causes of sudden death in the young. Hypertrophic cardiomyopathy, characterized by hypertrophy, myocyte disarray, and interstitial fibrosis, has been associated with mutations in sarcomeric genes. Patients who have hypertrophic cardiomyopathy and a mutation in the troponin T gene are at increased risk for sudden cardiac death despite a relatively mild degree of hypertrophy. In addition, patients who have specific mutations in the beta myosin heavy chain gene are also at greater risk for sudden cardiac death. These genotype–phenotype relationships impact clinical screening strategies and genetic counseling. Long QT syndrome, characterized by prolonged ventricular repolarization and ventricular tachycardia, has been associated with multiple genes, the vast majority of cases attributable to mutations in one of three ion channel genes. Patients who have long QT syndrome and mutations in either the KCNH2 or SCN5A genes seem to be at increased risk for cardiac events, impacting counseling and potentially decision making regarding the placement of an implantable cardioverter defibrillator. As medicine increasingly moves from diagnosis and treatment to screening and prevention, the family history plays an expanding role in clinical decision making. For example, all first-degree relatives of index cases who have hypertrophic cardiomyopathy or long QT syndrome may obtain genetic testing and if positive then undergo more aggressive clinical surveillance or intervention in an effort to prevent sudden cardiac death before any sign of disease. Many genetic diagnoses require comprehensive care and outcomes are improved by early coordination of care and early intervention. This approach shifts the emphasis from treating end-stage disease to treating anticipated disease.

Genetic screening for pediatric heart disease: an example

Family history also has a central role in the understanding of pediatric heart disease. Pediatric heart disease can be defined as cardiovascular disease in the young, including cardiovascular malformations (CVMs, also known as congenital heart defects), arrhythmias, cardiomyopathies, and vasculopathies. Pediatric heart disease is present in approximately 7 per 100 live births, and if one considers fetal abnormalities that result in spontaneous abortion before live birth, the incidence of CVM is at least five times higher [33,34]. Although an association between CVM and genetic syndromes has been established, the appreciation of single gene defects as a cause of nonsyndromic CVM has increased substantially in recent years. More than 1000 gene tests are now clinically available, including many for CVM in the context of a genetic syndrome; however, genetic testing for nonsyndromic CVM is primarily available on a research basis at this time (see http://www.genetests.org) [35,36].

Using the genetic family history in research

The working genetics research paradigm

Historically, genetic information was primarily ascertained from monogenic disorders that have unambiguous phenotypes and follow classic mendelian inheritance and account for approximately 5% of all disease; however, genetic information is rapidly being applied in novel ways to enhance diagnosis, risk stratification, and treatment in common complex diseases. The family history remains at the center of these efforts. Human genetic studies depend on precise and accurate phenotyping. Investigators appreciate that anything less, particularly in control groups, imposes major limitations in data analysis [37]. Despite thoroughly evaluating presumably normal participants, there are some factors that cannot be controlled. For example, at the time of evaluation, there is no way to know whether the individual is normal or simply has not manifested disease yet. In so far as it is possible, strict and narrow phenotype criteria facilitate accurate individual classification. Careful phenotyping is paramount once genetic cause is established and genotype–phenotype relationships can be elucidated.

The current paradigm in human genetics research involves genetic discovery (the identification of sequence variation associated with disease) followed by mechanistic investigation of the sequence variation in genetically modified animal models. Findings from human genetic studies are being taken into the laboratory where increasingly sophisticated animal models are providing the basis to define pathogenesis in various diseases. The elucidation of pathogenesis in turn results in the development of new diagnostic and therapeutic strategies, which can then be taken back to the patient. Taken together, this is referred to as the "bedside-to-bench-to-bedside" approach to disease and has led to numerous initiatives aiming to realize translational research goals. The Human Genome Project has reported the entire human sequence [38,39], and this achievement will facilitate the search for disease-causing genes and important sequence variation involved in the pathogenesis of complex diseases. Genetic information is also impacting the understanding of pharmacology as it relates to drug indications and drug responses, further facilitating improved care. Taken together, genetic information provides an impetus to shift the focus of medicine from treatment of end-stage disease to strategies emphasizing primary prevention and early intervention.

Hypoplastic left heart syndrome: an example

To illustrate how a detailed family history may be obtained and completed, the methods of an ongoing family-based study are described. A human genetics study is currently enrolling families identified by an index case who has hypoplastic left heart syndrome (HLHS) to identify the genetic causes of HLHS and associated CVM. HLHS (MIM#241550) is a severe CVM that continues to be a significant cause of infant mortality and childhood morbidity. Left-sided congenital CVMs, such as bicuspid aortic valve (BAV, MIM109730), aortic coarctation, and HLHS are believed to be causally related based on epidemiology studies that found familial clustering of these lesions. To date, more than 50 families have been recruited and nearly 250 family members have been evaluated. More than half of these families have at least one individual who has CVM in addition to the index case, demonstrating that these families are enriched for CVM. When a family is recruited, a detailed family history (minimum three generations) is obtained. A sequential sampling strategy is used (ie, each index case's first-degree relatives are evaluated and for every new affected individual identified, all of that person's first-degree relatives are evaluated). When the family history identifies a second-degree relative who is affected, all of that person's first-degree relatives are evaluated. Each family member who is evaluated undergoes phlebotomy for

DNA analysis and an echocardiogram for evaluation of cardiac anatomy. All family members undergo echocardiographic screening even if they are otherwise healthy. Careful phenotyping is critical because BAV often is subclinical.

Family history was reviewed with at least two family members on at least three separate occasions. In 28 of 38 (74%) kindreds, the initial family history was not altered by subsequent inquiries. In 10 of 38 (26%) families, however, information relevant to the study was either revised or discovered on subsequent queries and in all instances led to the discovery of a multiplex kindred. In 4 of 10 (40%) of these families, significant revisions on multiple occasions were necessary to arrive at a complete family history.

For example, the family represented in Fig. 1 shows the development of family history information. The index case (individual IV-1, indicated by an arrowhead) was diagnosed at birth and transferred to a cardiac intensive care unit for further care. On admission, the family history was taken from the father and noted to be noncontributory. During the course of the hospitalization, the family was approached to invite participation in the human genetics study. At that time a detailed family history was obtained from the mother and it was discovered that the maternal great-grandmother (I-2) had a history of BAV and aortic valve disease requiring aortic valve replacement, underscoring the importance of talking with different people within the same family to gather all relevant information. Medical records, including imaging reports and operative reports, were obtained to confirm the family history and document specific medical details. Subsequently, two previously unknown cases of BAV were identified by screening echocardiography in the father (III-1) and a sibling (IV-2). The discovery of subclinical CVM highlights the importance of careful phenotyping and screening first-degree relatives at risk (individuals who have BAV are at increased risk for developing aortic valve disease, infective endocarditis, and aortic root dissection). The mother (III-2) and maternal grandfather (II-3) are obligate carriers and therefore presumably have the genotype associated with disease without any evidence of the phenotype. Taken together, pedigree analysis of this family is consistent with autosomal recessive inheritance and reduced penetrance.

HLHS and associated CVM have a heritability of 74%, suggesting that HLHS is caused largely by genetic factors [40]. This high heritability predicts that areas of the genome can be mapped

---

Box 2. Summary: take-home messages

A detailed family history is necessary for optimal clinical use and research.
The family history must be obtained from multiple family members on different occasions.
The "complete" family history must be revisited regularly.
The pedigree is a useful tool for consolidating medical information and patient education.
There are informative and useful Web-based resources for patients and health care
    providers.
The family history is critical to the continued success of human genetics research.
The family history may indicate genetic screening, which in turn may direct medical care.

---

and disease-causing genes identified, which in turn may lead to the development of genetically modified animal models of HLHS and an improved understanding of pathogenesis. Ultimately, this may lead to new strategies directed at diagnosis and treatment. A better understanding of the genetic basis of HLHS may refine the way we think about CVM. The current taxonomy of CVM is based on anatomy, and it is unclear how genetic insight may improve our understanding of the clinical taxonomy.

The frequency of first-degree relatives who have HLHS or CVM is approximately 3% and 18%. Siblings of HLHS index cases were diagnosed with HLHS in 8% of cases and any CVM in 22% of cases. Recurrence risk ratios for first-degree relatives and siblings were significantly increased. If one parent was affected with CVM, the frequency and recurrence risk ratios of siblings who had either HLHS or CVM increased substantially [40]. This finding suggests that epidemiology-based recurrence risk calculations underestimate risk, possibly because of incomplete phenotyping of first-degree relatives, and this should be taken into consideration when counseling families.

A strength of this approach is the use of a strict phenotype definition of HLHS and precise echocardiographic phenotyping. Human genetic studies depend on careful and accurate phenotyping. Left ventricular hypoplasia, a feature of several different CVMs (eg, unbalanced atrioventricular septal defect) believed to have diverse developmental origins, is often referred to as HLHS based in part on the similarity of the surgical treatment strategy of individuals who have a left ventricular hypoplasia. This similarity results in the generic use of "HLHS" in the literature, which is problematic when considering the genetic basis of HLHS. Combining echocardiography, which obtains detailed and definitive phenotype information, with a narrow, well-defined index case

definition provides consistent and specific results. Our findings also demonstrate the benefit of a thorough detailed family history in human genetics research, and emphasize the need to revisit the family history vigilantly and the medical value of family history awareness.

Summary

Genetics has transformed the use of family history information and has led to the reemergence of the detailed genetic family history (Box 2). It is critical that public and professional educational efforts to increase family history awareness and working knowledge are prioritized. Patient maintenance of the pedigree provides increased patient awareness and facilitates some of the limitations associated with conventional medical history ascertainment, ultimately improving health care and research. Detailed family history information is superior to abbreviated family history information, and detailed family histories are necessary for the optimal use of genetic screening. The increasing use of genetic screening promises to cultivate a paradigm shift in medical treatment emphasizing primary prevention and early intervention. Appreciation of the family history is necessary to make this important advance.

References

[1] Fielding G. History of medicine. New York (NY): WB Saunders Company; 1966.
[2] Bennett R. The practical guide to the genetic family history. Wilmington (DE): Wiley-Liss, Inc.; 1999.
[3] Guttmacher AE, Collins FS, Carmona RH. The family history—more important than ever. N Engl J Med 2004;351(22):2333–6.
[4] Yoon PW, Scheuner MT, Peterson-Oehlke KL, et al. Can family history be used as a tool for public health and preventive medicine? Genet Med 2002;4(4): 304–10.

[5] Kirkham C, Harris S, Grzybowski S. Evidence-based prenatal care: part I. General prenatal care and counseling issues. Am Fam Physician 2005;71(7):1307–16.

[6] Mendel G. Experiments in plant hybridization. Journal of the Royal Horticultural Society 1901;26:1–32.

[7] Tools G. SCREEN for familial disease. Available at: www.genetests.org. Accessed October 23, 2007.

[8] Clarke J. A clinical guide to inherited metabolic diseases. New York (NY): Cambridge University Press; 1996.

[9] Coonar AS, McKenna WJ. Molecular genetics of familial cardiomyopathies. Adv Genet 1997;35: 285–324.

[10] Bennett RL, Hampel HL, Mandell JB, et al. Genetic counselors: translating genomic science into clinical practice. J Clin Invest 2003;112(9):1274–9.

[11] Barlow-Stewart K, Gaff G, Emery J, et al. Family genetics. Aust Fam Physician 2007;36(10):802–5.

[12] Bennett RL. The family medical history. Prim Care 2004;31(3):479–95.

[13] Scheuner MT, Wang SJ, Raffel LJ, et al. Family history: a comprehensive genetic risk assessment method for the chronic conditions of adulthood. Am J Med Genet 1997;71(3):315–24.

[14] Williams RR, Hunt SC, Heiss G, et al. Usefulness of cardiovascular family history data for population-based preventive medicine and medical research (the Health Family Tree Study and the NHLBI Family Heart Study). Am J Cardiol 2001;87(2):129–35.

[15] Rich EC, Burke W, Heaton CJ, et al. Reconsidering the family history in primary care. J Gen Intern Med 2004;19(3):273–80.

[16] Trotter TL, Martin HM. Family history in pediatric primary care. Pediatrics 2007;120(Suppl 2):S60–5.

[17] Bennett RL, Steinhaus KA, Uhrich SB, et al. Recommendations for standardized human pedigree nomenclature. Pedigree standardization task force of the National Society of Genetic Counselors. Am J Hum Genet 1995;56(3):745–52.

[18] Ciarleglio LJ, Bennet RL, Williamson J, et al. Genetic counseling throughout the life cycle. J Clin Invest 2003;112(9):1280–6.

[19] Collins FS, Bochm K. Avoiding casualties in the genetic revolution: the urgent need to educate physicians about genetics. Acad Med 1999;74(1):48–9.

[20] Acheson LS, Weisner GL, Zyzonski SJ, et al. Family history-taking in community family practice: implications for genetic screening. Genet Med 2000;2(3): 180–5.

[21] Walter FM, Emery J. "Coming down the line"—patients' understanding of their family history of common chronic disease. Ann Fam Med 2005;3(5): 405–14.

[22] Chessa M, DeRosa G, Pardeo M, et al. What do parents know about the malformations afflicting the hearts of their children? Cardiol Young 2005;15(2):125–9.

[23] Frezzo TM, Rubistein WS, Dunham D, et al. The genetic family history as a risk assessment tool in internal medicine. Genet Med 2003;5(2):84–91.

[24] Greendale K, Pyeritz RE. Empowering primary care health professionals in medical genetics: how soon? How fast? How far? Am J Med Genet 2001;106(3): 223–32.

[25] Jenkins J, Grady PA, Collins FS. Nurses and the genomic revolution. J Nurs Scholarsh 2005;37(2): 98–101.

[26] Romitti PA. Utility of family history reports of major birth defects as a public health strategy. Pediatrics 2007;120(Suppl 2):S71–7.

[27] Almasy L, Blangero J. Multipoint quantitative-trait linkage analysis in general pedigrees. Am J Hum Genet 1998;62(5):1198–211.

[28] Benson DW, Sharkey A, Fatkin D, et al. Reduced penetrance, variable expressivity, and genetic heterogeneity of familial atrial septal defects. Circulation 1998;97(20):2043–9.

[29] Hinton RB, Yutzey KE, Benson DW. Congenital heart disease: genetic causes and developmental insights. Prog Pediatr Cardiol 2005;20:101–11.

[30] Kardia SL, Modell SM, Peyser PA. Family-centered approaches to understanding and preventing coronary heart disease. Am J Prev Med 2003;24(2): 143–51.

[31] Crouch MA, Gramling R. Family history of coronary heart disease: evidence-based applications. Prim Care 2005;32(4):995–1010.

[32] Harmon A. Cancer free at 33, but weighing a mastectomy. N Y Times, September 16, 2007. Available at: www.nytimes.com/2007/09/16/health/16gene.html.

[33] Hoffman JI, Kaplan S. The incidence of congenital heart disease. J Am Coll Cardiol 2002;39(12): 1890–900.

[34] Hoffman JI. Incidence of congenital heart disease: II. Prenatal incidence. Pediatr Cardiol 1995;16(4): 155–65.

[35] Pierpont ME, Basson CT, Benson DW, et al. Genetic basis for congenital heart defects: current knowledge: a scientific statement from the American Heart Association Congenital Cardiac Defects Committee, Council on Cardiovascular Disease in the Young: endorsed by the American Academy of Pediatrics. Circulation 2007;115(23):3015–38.

[36] Robin NH, Tabereaux PB, Benza R, et al. Genetic testing in cardiovascular disease. J Am Coll Cardiol 2007;50(8):727–37.

[37] Luo AK, Jefferson BK, Garcia MJ, et al. Challenges in the phenotypic characterisation of patients in genetic studies of coronary artery disease. J Med Genet 2007;44(3):161–5.

[38] Venter JC, Adams MD, Myers EW, et al. The sequence of the human genome. Science 2001; 291(5507):1304–51.

[39] Lander ES, Linton LM, Birren B, et al. Initial sequencing and analysis of the human genome. Nature 2001;409(6822):860–921.

[40] Hinton RB Jr, Martin LJ, Tabangin ME, et al. Hypoplastic left heart syndrome is heritable. J Am Coll Cardiol 2007;50(16):1590–5.

ELSEVIER
SAUNDERS

Crit Care Nurs Clin N Am 20 (2008) 159–169

CRITICAL CARE
NURSING CLINICS
OF NORTH AMERICA

Congenital Heart Disease and Genetics

Vicki L. Zeigler, PhD, RN

College of Nursing, Texas Woman's University, P.O. Box 425498, Denton, TX 76204-5498, USA

Congenital heart disease (CHD) refers to "any abnormality in circulatory structure or function that is present at birth, even if it is discovered much later" [1]. The true incidence of CHD is elusive in that most calculations do not include bicuspid aortic valves, mitral valve prolapse, or congenital rhythm and conduction problems, such as long QT syndrome and complete atrioventricular block; however, an analytic review of published studies [2] reports the incidence of moderate to severe forms of CHD as approximately 6 per 1000 live births (which increases to 19 per 1000 live births if serious bicuspid aortic valves are included). If all forms of CHD, including tiny muscular ventricular septal defects (VSDs) present at birth and other trivial lesions, are included the incidence increases to 74 per 1000 live births [2,3].

The cause of CHD is both genetic and environmental [4]. Although the field of genetics remains in its infancy, information regarding the genetic basis of CHD is expanding rapidly and experts believe that it has been considerably underestimated in the past [5]. The purpose of this discussion is to identify what is currently known about the genetic basis of CHD. First, common congenital heart defects are discussed by anatomic category, including septal defects, obstructive lesions, and complex cardiovascular malformations. Second, genetic and chromosomal syndromes with associated cardiac defects are described. Third, the genetics of congenital cardiac arrhythmias are presented followed by the nursing considerations, including available genetic testing.

Septal defects

Atrial septal defects (ASDs), VSDs, and atrioventricular septal defects are lesions that produce left-to-right shunting. Atrial septal defects account for approximately 10% of all congenital heart defects [6] and are described according to their location: (a) sinus venosus defect, (b) ostium secundum defect, and (c) ostium primum defect. Atrial septal defects can be found in patients who have certain syndromes, including Holt-Oram, Ellis–van Creveld, and Noonan syndromes.

The inheritance patterns of ASDs were studied as early as the 1960s [7,8], at which time it was believed that ASDs were attributable to mutations a single major gene. Three families of multiple generations were studied and although the most common anomaly was ASD, other defects occurred alone or in association with ASD in individuals from each kindred. In one kindred, the researchers were able to localize a familial ASD gene to 5p [9]. In 1998, Benson and colleagues provided evidence that there was reduced penetrance (fewer than 100% of people who have the genotype have the phenotype), variable expressivity (people who have the same genotype have differences in severity of affectedness), and genetic heterogeneity (the same phenotype is produced by several gene variants) of familial ASDs [9].

Several transcription factors have been associated with familial ASD. Familial ASD with progressive atrioventricular block (AVB) is autosomal dominant and is associated with mutations or haploinsufficiency of the NKX2.5 gene on chromosome 5 [5]. The secundum ASD associated with Holt-Oram syndrome is autosomal dominant, has variable expression, and results from mutations of the TBX5 gene on 12q24.1. Familial ASD without progressive AVB is associated with GATA 4 mutations [10].

VSDs are the most common congenital cardiac lesion, accounting for 40% of all congenital heart defects [2]. VSDs are classified according to their location and include the following: (a)

E-mail address: vzeigler@twu.edu

perimembranous, (b) muscular, (c) inlet, and (d) subpulmonary. VSDs are associated with deletions or duplications in several chromosomes, including trisomies 13, 18, and 21 [5]. VSDs can be present in children who have Holt-Oram syndrome in addition to nine other syndromes [5].

Atrioventricular septal defect (AVSD), also referred to as endocardial cushion defect (ECD) or AV canal defect, accounts for 5% of congenital cardiac defects [2] and occurs as a result of the failure of atrial and ventricular septation. If the defect is complete, an ostium primum ASD is present that is combined with an inlet defect within the ventricular septum with a single inlet valve replacing the mitral and tricuspid valves. Sixty percent of children born with this cardiac defect have Down syndrome or trisomy 21 [5]. Isolated AVSDs are inherited as autosomal dominant traits with a gene locus mapped to 1p31p21. There is variable expression and incomplete penetrance. In a successive series of 103 isolated AVSDs (ie, not associated with trisomy 21 or other syndromes) Digilio and colleagues [11] reported the likelihood of relatives of a proband being affected. The risks were a 3.6% chance for siblings, a 1.9% chance for the parents, and a 0.8% chance for aunts and uncles. AVSDs have been mapped to two genes, AVSD1 and AVSD2. Sheffield and colleagues [12] screened the genomes in an extended kindred and identified a genetic locus on chromosome 1 shared by all affected individuals. They found a congenital heart defect susceptibility gene variant, inherited as an autosomal dominant trait with incomplete penetrance. The genetic map locus for AVSD was identified as chromosome 1p31-p21.

Obstructive lesions

The three major congenital cardiac lesions that pose obstruction to blood flow include pulmonary stenosis (PS), aortic stenosis (AS), and coarctation of the aorta (CoA). In children who have PS, pulmonary blood flow is obstructed, and in children who have AS and CoA, systemic blood flow is obstructed.

Pulmonary stenosis

Pulmonary stenosis is responsible for approximately 10% of CHD [2] and is simply a narrowing into the pulmonary artery that interferes with blood flow from the right ventricle. This narrowing can occur at the valve level (valvular PS), below the valve (subvalvular PS), or above the

valve (supravalvular PS), and several areas of stenosis may occur simultaneously. Pulmonary valve stenosis is associated with several syndromes, including Noonan, Alagille, Costello, and LEOPARD syndromes, along with other chromosomal abnormalities.

Aortic stenosis

Aortic stenosis (AS) is a narrowing into the aorta and occurs in 5% to 10% of all CHD. This narrowing causes an obstruction to blood flow from the left ventricle and may occur at the following levels: valvular, subvalvular, or supravalvular, with valvular AS being the most common. Aortic valve stenosis is also associated with Noonan and Turner syndromes. Studies regarding the familial basis of supravalvular AS (SVAS) began in the 1960s [13,14]. Frequently associated with Williams syndrome, it was initially believed to be a part of that syndrome's contiguous gene deletion; however, in 1993, Curran and colleagues [15] reported a family who had autosomal dominant SVAS. They identified a translocation that cosegregated with the disease and also disrupted the elastin gene, with a breakpoint that localized to exon 28 of the gene. It was then mapped to 7q11.2 [16] and others confirmed through further studies that SVAS was indeed linked to the elastin gene [17].

Bicuspid aortic valve

Bicuspid aortic valve (BAV) occurs in 1% of the population, yet is often omitted in the estimation of the incidence of CHD. BAV commonly precedes the development of aortic valve insufficiency or aortic stenosis and has recently been identified as having an almost entirely genetic basis. In their study of 309 probands who had BAV and their relatives, Cripe and colleagues [18] found a prevalence of 24% for BAV (n = 74) and a prevalence of 31% for BAV or other cardiovascular malformations (n = 97), with a heritability of BAV alone of 89% and of BAV and other cardiovascular malformations of 75%. They concluded that this heritability suggested that valve malformation can be primary to defective valvulogenesis or secondary to other elements of cardiogenesis.

Coarctation of the aorta

Coarctation of the aorta is a narrowing of the aorta that impedes systemic blood flow and occurs in 10% of children who have CHD. The narrowing in CoA is generally beyond the left subclavian artery at the location of the ductus arteriosus; however, it may occur in locations proximal or distal to this site also. Approximately 50% of children who have CoA also have a bicuspid aortic valve. Familial CoA was initially described in a father and son in 1961 [19]. In the mid 1980s, researchers described the defect in four generations [20]. Recently Leffredo and colleagues [21] studied the families of 46 probands who had CoA. Their sample also included 38 probands who had hypoplastic left heart and 22 probands who had transposition of the great arteries, with the latter being used as controls. It was this study that confirmed the familial aggregation of CoA with a more frequent occurrence in first-degree relatives (9.4%), followed by less than 1% in second-degree relatives and 1.2% in third-degree relatives. Most of the cardiovascular lesions were left-sided obstructive lesions [21].

CoA is considered one of several left ventricular outflow tract obstructions (LVOTO). The other defects placed in this category include hypoplastic left heart/ventricle, aortic valve stenosis, bicuspid aortic valve, and hypoplastic aortic arch. By examining these disorders as a group, Wessels and colleagues [22] suggested that LVOTO lesions are related developmentally and may occasionally be caused by a single-gene defect. A large study of 124 families who had LVOTO lesions found a heritability rate of 17.7% (32 of 413 relatives) of LVOTO lesions and other significant heart defects. The researchers concluded that the relative risk for first-degree relatives was 36.9%, which supported the notion that two or more genes are probably working together to produce the phenotype [23].

Complex cardiovascular malformations

Complex cardiovascular malformations in which there is right-to-left shunting are often referred to as cyanotic defects. Children who have cyanotic defects may experience increased or decreased pulmonary blood flow depending on the specific lesion. A discussion of all of the congenital cardiac cyanotic defects is beyond the scope of this article; however, four of these defects warrant discussion. They include tetralogy of Fallot (TOF), transposition of the great arteries (TGA), truncus arteriosus (TA), and hypoplastic left heart syndrome (HLHS).

Tetralogy of Fallot

Tetralogy of Fallot is the most common cyanotic defect and accounts for 9% to 14% of all CHD. Four anomalies make up TOF, including a VSD, an overriding aorta, PS, and right ventricular hypertrophy. This defect may occur in conjunction with other abnormalities and the degree of right-to-left shunting varies with the amount of PS and the degree of right ventricular outflow obstruction, with moderate pulmonary obstruction producing elevated right ventricular pressures. Inheritance patterns of TOF have been studied for more than 40 years. There is now a documented association with 22q11 microdeletion [24,25]. In 1999 Benson and colleagues reported that mutations in the cardiac transcription factor NKX 2.5 altered cardiac development [26].

In 2001, a missense mutation (G274D) in JAG 1 was identified (JAG1 mutations cause Alagille syndrome) in a large kindred of autosomal dominant TOF with reduced penetrance [27]. Nine of the 11 carriers had manifest cardiac defects, including standard TOF, VSD with TGA, and isolated peripheral PS. Although none of the individuals in this kindred met the diagnostic criteria for any syndrome, all forms of TOF were represented, including associated PS/atresia and the absence of the pulmonary valve [27].

In this same year, Goldmuntz and colleagues [28] studied 114 patients who had TOF and no evidence of a 22q11 microdeletion. Four mutations in the transcription factor NKX2.5 were identified in 6 of the study participants who had the following diagnoses: 3 had standard TOF with varying anatomies of the aortic arch, and the remainder had pulmonary valve atresia with or without major aortopulmonary collateral vessels. Although only 1 individual had a family history of TOF, several other participants were found to be asymptomatic carriers, suggesting reduced penetrance.

Transposition of the great arteries

Transposition of the great arteries (dextro-TGA or simply d-TGA) is a cyanotic defect that occurs in 10% to 11% of children who have CHD. Also known as complete transposition, with d-TGA, the aorta arises from the right ventricle (versus the proper left ventricle) and the pulmonary artery arises from the left ventricle (versus the proper right ventricle). The transposed arteries result in unoxygenated blood entering from the right atrium, continuing to the right ventricle, and out of the aorta into systemic recirculation. Oxygenated blood enters the left atrium, continues to the left ventricle, and through the pulmonary artery to recirculate through the pulmonary system. This process results in two separate circulations and mixing of oxygenated blood with unoxygenated blood cannot occur without the presence of a VSD, an ASD, a patent foramen ovale (PFO), or a patent ductus arteriosus (PDA) [29].

The frequency of cardiac defects in first-degree relatives of probands who had TGA was first reported in 1996 [29]. The 271 study participants or probands were divided into four groups: levo-TGA (l-TGA), d-TGA, complex TGA, and TGA with asplenia with 19, 168, 65, and 19 individuals per group, respectively. In the d-TGA group, there were 369 siblings of which only one had a cardiac defect (0.27%). In the l-TGA group, only one of the 50 siblings had a cardiac defect (2.0%), and in the complex TGA group, 2 of 143 (1.4%) had cardiac defects. Last, in the group with TGA and asplenia, 1 of 50 (2.0%) of the siblings had a cardiac defect. The researchers concluded that the overall risk for recurrence in the siblings of probands who had TGA was 0.82%. A parental occurrence rate of 0.55% was calculated based on the percentage of malformation found in each group: 0.29% in the d-TGA group, 0% in the l-TGA group, 1.54% in the complex TGA group, and 0% for the TGA with asplenia group [29].

In 2002, Goldmuntz and colleagues [30] identified a mutation in the CFC1 gene in patients who had TGA and double-outlet right ventricle. Two disease-related mutations were found in 86 patients and were identified as autosomal single-gene defects, indicating the pivotal role that CFC1 plays in the development of the cardiovascular system [30]. Muncke and colleagues [31] identified a de novo (not seen before in the family) balanced chromosomal translocation 46,XX,t(12,17) (q24.1q21) in a 7-year-old girl who had TGA (with a perimembranous VSD, PFO, and mild CoA) and mental retardation. Further genetic testing revealed a variation in a novel gene, PROSIT240. This case study prompted screening of an additional 97 patients who had TGA for these mutations, which led to the identification of three missense mutations that change amino acids.

Truncus arteriosus

TA is defined as an outflow tract defect and it occurs when the conotruncal area does not divide and separate during fetal cardiac development into a separate aorta and pulmonary artery, resulting in a common trunk that supplies arterial, systemic, and coronary artery circulations. Infants who have TA have a common valve referred to as a truncal valve instead of two separate pulmonary and aortic valves. Families and their children who have conotruncal (outflow tract) abnormalities have been studied as early as 1988, when Pierpont and colleagues [32] established a higher recurrence risk for these types of defects compared with other cardiac defects and suggested a monogenic inheritance pattern. This study was followed by others that demonstrated a familial link to TA and other outflow tract defects [33,34].

Commonly associated with DiGeorge syndrome, the family of conotruncal defects account for one quarter to one third of all congenital heart defects not associated with a syndrome; however, many studies involving conotruncal defects are associated with what has become known as conotruncal anomaly face syndrome or CAFS [35–37]. Genetic findings to date include evidence that: (a) a mutation in the CFC1 plays a part in the origination of another conotruncal defect, namely double-outlet right ventricle, (b) mutations in the TBX1 gene may be related to the 22q11.2 deletion syndrome, which includes patients who have CAFS, and (c) a mutation in the GDF1 gene has been found to be associated with double-outlet right ventricle also [10].

Hypoplastic left heart syndrome

HLHS is a serious defect that accounts for 1% of all CHD. It is the most common cause of death in the first month of life in neonates who have CHD. The major defect in HLHS is a severely underdeveloped left ventricle. Blood enters the right side as normal, but from the right ventricle some blood goes to the lungs and some to the aorta by way of a right-to-left shunt across the PDA. Systemic blood is then supplied by way of the PDA. Pulmonary blood enters the left atrium and is shunted across the ASD/PFO into the right atrium.

It has been speculated since the 1970s that HLHS was a heritable congenital heart defect [38–40]. In 2004, Loffredo and colleages [21] identified 38 probands who had HLHS and their families, 46 who had CoA and 22 who had d-TGA. Cardiac anomalies were found more frequently in the first-degree relatives of probands who had HLHS (19.35%) or CoA (9.4%) than d-TGA families.

Less than 1% of second-degree relatives were affected in all three groups and for the third-degree relatives, cardiac anomalies occurred in 1.8% of families who had HLHS, 1.2% in families who had CoA, and 0.4% in families who had TGA.

Considered to be a member of the left ventricular outflow tract obstruction family, HLHS has been included in other genetic studies, including the other members of this defect's family (eg, CoA, AS, BAV). These studies suggested that HLHS is developmentally related and can be caused by a single-gene defect [22]. Recently, researchers have confirmed that HLHS is probably largely determined by genetic factors [41]. Hinton and colleagues have provided the first estimate of the heritability of HLHS using variance component methodology, indicating high heritability. Their sample included 38 probands who had HLHS and a three-generation family history. All of the probands had aortic valve dysplasia and other valve abnormalities were found, including the mitral valve in 94%, the tricuspid valve in 56%, and the pulmonary valve in 11%. More than one half (55%) of enrolled families had more than one affected individual. The heritability for HLHS was found to be 99% and for HLHS and associated cardiovascular malformations was 74%. The recurrence risk in siblings was 8% for HLHS alone and 22% for cardiovascular malformations [41,43]. Taken together, these findings suggested that HLHS is a severe form of valve malformation.

Genetic syndromes with a congenital heart disease component

There are many genetic syndromes and chromosomal abnormalities with a cardiac component and many children who have congenital heart defects have extracardiac malformations. Approximately 20% to 45% of children who have congenital heart defects have certain specific extracardiac abnormalities [42,43]. Although the number of genetic syndromes and chromosomal abnormalities are beyond the scope of this discussion, three of the most common syndromes with associated cardiac defects are described.

Down syndrome (trisomy 21)

Many chromosomal disorders have associated cardiac anomalies. The most familiar of these is trisomy 21 or Down syndrome. Approximately 95% of all infants who have Down syndrome have trisomy 21 due to nondisjunction [44] and

the most common structural malformations in these infants are cardiac [45].

Children who have Down syndrome have an upward outward slant of the palpebral fissure and epicanthic folds across the inside corners of the eyes. Other noncardiac features found in newborns who have Down syndrome include hypotonia, decreased Moro reflex with hyperextensibility of the joints, a flat facial profile, excess skin around the back of the neck, and small ears that may be decreased in length and may be round or square in appearance [45]. Half of infants who have Down syndrome have palmar creases of their hands and the degree to which the child is mentally retarded varies [45].

The incidence of associated heart disease in children who have Down syndrome has been reported as high as 70%, but it is probably closer to 40% to 50% [46]. Although individuals who have trisomy 21 can have tetralogy of Fallot or transposition of the great arteries, the most common defect associated with Down syndrome is AVSD, also known as endocardial cushion defect. It occurs in 60% of cases; however, ASDs and VSDs are also common [46].

Noonan syndrome

Noonan syndrome was first described in 1963 by Noonan and Ehmke [42] who reported nine patients who had valvular pulmonary stenosis, short stature, mild mental retardation, hypotelorism, and unusual facial features. Noonan syndrome is estimated to occur in 1 in 1000 to 1 in 2500 live births [47]. Other noncardiac features characteristic of Noonan's syndrome include broad or webbed neck, unusual chest shape, characteristic facies, developmental delay, and cryptorchidism [5].

Approximately two thirds of patients who have Noonan syndrome have some type of cardiac defect, half of which are valvar pulmonic stenosis [47,48]. It is an autosomal dominant trait and 25% to 70% of cases result from de novo mutations [5]. In addition to being associated with pulmonary valve stenosis, Noonan syndrome is also associated with hypertrophic cardiomyopathy. Mutations in several genes (PTPN11, KAAS, and SOS1) are responsible for Noonan syndrome.

DiGeorge syndrome

DiGeorge syndrome was first described in 1953 as a combination of thymic hypoplasia, parathyroid hypoplasia, and cardiac defects [49].

Children who have DiGeorge syndrome experience persistent hypocalcemia and their parathyroid glands may be absent or reduced in size and number. The thymus may be absent, small, or ectopic, and some of these children have minor facial abnormalities. The two most common cardiac defects associated with DiGeorge syndrome are conotruncal defects, such as truncus arteriosus, and branchial arch mesenchymal tissue defects (eg, interrupted aortic arch) [50]. Additional conotruncal defects associated with DiGeorge syndrome include tetralogy of Fallot with or without absent pulmonary valve syndrome, pulmonary atresia, interrupted aortic arch type B, or right aortic arch. Other congenital cardiac defects associated with DiGeorge syndrome include TGA, HLHS, and aberrant left subclavian artery.

DiGeorge syndrome can result from chromosomal abnormalities and single-gene defects (transmitted in autosomal dominant or autosomal recessive patterns) [51] and from teratogenic exposures and in association with other defects [45]. Most children who have DiGeorge syndrome are born with a deletion of chromosome 22q11, leading to the syndrome's nickname, Catch-22 [52].

Congenital cardiac arrhythmias

Cardiac arrhythmias in the young are often attributable to a genetic defect. Although the gene variant is present at birth, its results may not be seen early in life; however, these abnormalities in cardiac rhythm and conduction are considered congenital heart problems. Probably the first genetic cardiac defect identified as a congenital arrhythmia was QT prolongation in children who were deaf [53]. The subsequently named long QT syndrome (LQTS) is one of the more common and variable of the congenital arrhythmia syndromes. The same gene mutation in the same family may result in sudden death of an infant, sudden death associated with athletics, or the absence of symptoms over the lifespan. This variation in penetrance and expressivity is not well understood, but because the LQTS is attributable to abnormalities in cardiac ion channels and adaptor proteins, it can be postulated that other genes controlling membrane proteins affect the channels also [54].

Long QT syndrome

LQTS is a genetically determined abnormality of ventricular repolarization that results in cardiac

instability that can lead to life-threatening arrhythmias or sudden death. This potentially lethal cardiac arrhythmia is responsible for 3000 to 4000 sudden deaths in children and young adults each year in the United States [55]. The diagnosis of LQTS relies on presentation of a group of clinical and ECG manifestations along with prolongation of the QT interval. Clinical signs in children and adolescents can include the following: syncope (associated with noise, stress, or exercise), presyncope, palpitations, seizures, ventricular arrhythmias, cardiac arrest, or sudden death. Associated findings may include congenital AV block, congenital deafness (rare), syndactyly (rare), and a family history of LQTS or sudden death.

LQTS was originally characterized by Jervell and Lange-Nielsen [53] in 1957 as a recessively transmitted syndrome involving congenital deafness, prolonged QT, and the potentially lethal ventricular arrhythmia, torsade de pointes. Romano and colleagues in 1963 [56] and Ward in 1964 [57] described the characteristics of prolonged QT/torsade de pointes, syncope/sudden death, and an autosomal dominant inheritance pattern. In 1997, researchers determined that mutations in the KCNQ1 (KVLQT1) gene were a cause of the autosomal dominant form of Romano Ward syndrome and the recessive form of Jervell and Lange-Nielsen syndrome [58]. In 1991, Keating and colleagues [59] reported that LQTS resulted from sodium and potassium ion channel abnormalities caused by abnormal proteins encoded by mutated genes.

LQTS is caused by genetically defined defects in potassium, sodium, or calcium channels in cardiac cells. To date, more than 300 mutations have been identified in genes encoding key ion channel subunits and adapter proteins involved in the organization of the heart's action potential [60]. The three phenotypes that compose most of the cases include LQT1 (50%), LQT2 (35%–45%), and LQT3 (3%–15%), with the remainder accounting for less than 1% of cases [55].

Linkage analysis studies for LQTS accelerated in the 1990s and resulted in the mapping of four loci for LQTS on three chromosomes: chromosome 11, chromosome 3, and chromosome 7 [61]. LQT1, the most ubiquitous form of congenital LQTS, results from mutations in the KCNQ1 (KVLQT1) gene affecting the function of a cardiac potassium channel. In a study using data from the International LQTS Registry, Locati and colleagues [62] assessed 479 probands and found that the first cardiac event associated with LQTS occurred significantly earlier in males and this effect was more pronounced in carriers of a KCNQ1 (KVLQT1) mutation Clinically, individuals who have LQT1 have an increased risk for having an arrhythmic event during physical exercise, particularly swimming [63].

LQT2, the second most common form of congenital LQTS, is caused by mutations in a potassium channel gene, specifically the KCNH2 gene located on chromosome 7, which results in a reduction in the potassium current and subsequent delayed repolarization [61]. Clinically, individuals who have LQT2 are at an increased risk for lethal cardiac events during emotional stress and also are at risk during sleep and at rest. Interestingly, 80% of events in patients who have LQT2 are related to auditory stimuli [63]. LQT3 is attributable to mutations in the cardiac sodium channel gene SCN5A, which is located on chromosome 3. The prevalence of this type of LQTS is believed to be in the range of 10% to 15% [61]. Clinically, patients who have LQT3 experience most of their cardiac events at rest or while sleeping (64%). Only 4% of these patients will experience an event during exercise [63].

Numerous additional genes have been implicated in LQTS, some occurring within syndromes (Anderson and Timothy syndromes) and some causing isolated QT prolongation [61].

Brugada syndrome

Brugada syndrome (BrS) is a cardiac channelopathy. In the late 1980s, six cases were described in which the patients experienced ventricular fibrillation and unusual ST segment morphology elevation along with a right bundle branch block pattern on their ECGs [64]. In 1992, the Brugada brothers [65] described an additional eight patients who experienced sudden cardiac arrest and who had the same ECG characteristics as those described by Martini and colleagues in the 1980 article. The combination of the ECG characteristics of right bundle branch block and ST segment elevation coupled with sudden death was named Brugada syndrome [65].

Missense mutations in the sodium channel gene (SCN5A) gene have been found in individuals who have Brugada syndrome [66]. In a study of 130 probands who had BrS, Priori and colleagues [67] identified SCN5A mutations in 28. In 2002, Weiss and colleagues [68] reported that 12 members of a multigenerational family demonstrated an autosomal dominant pattern of inheritance with incomplete penetrance. Linkages to chromosome 3 were found leading the researchers to conclude that there is a locus distinct from SCN5A in individuals who have BrS. Like LQTS, several genes have been implicated, but because BrS is rare the relative frequency of involvement is unclear [68].

Catecholaminergic polymorphic ventricular tachycardia

Catecholaminergic polymorphic ventricular tachycardia (CPVT) is an inherited syncope/sudden death syndrome resulting from abnormal handling of calcium by the sarcoplasmic reticulum. First described in 1978 [69] and again in 1995 [70], CPVT resulted in syncope in children and adolescents who had structurally normal hearts and normal QT intervals. CPVT is distinct from other forms of syncope in that it is stress related and consistently reproducible. It is also associated with sudden death.

Priori and colleagues [71] reported the first gene locus and suggested that the cardiac ryanodine receptor gene mapped to this locus may be responsible for CVPT. CPVT is caused by mutations in the genes RYR2 (ryanodine receptor) and CASQ2 (calsequestrin 2). The ryanodine receptor is a channel for calcium release from the sarcoplasmic reticulum into the cytosol where large amounts of calcium are stored [72,73].

Sick sinus syndrome

Sick sinus syndrome (SSS) is a broad term that describes arrhythmias resulting from abnormal sinus node function and includes a wide array of bradyarrhythmias, including sinus bradycardia, sinus pause/arrest, sinoatrial exit block, and slow escape rhythms, including junctional bradycardia. Although most commonly acquired during surgery for congenital heart disease that requires close proximity to the sinus node, SSS can be congenital. Mutations in the cardiac sodium channel gene SCN5A can result in congenital SSS [74].

Nursing considerations

Nurses caring for children who have genetic conditions are in a unique position and can be of great assistance to patients and families; nurses at the bedside may be the first to learn of a familial condition and a clear understanding of genetic evaluation, counseling, and testing is needed.

Genetic testing

There are available genetic tests for many syndromes that are strongly associated with structural CHD (eg, Noonan syndrome and associated pulmonary valve stenosis) and most chromosomal abnormalities are associated with CHD (eg, Down syndrome and complete AVSD). Although there may not be an available genetic test specifically for TOF, there is a genetic test for DiGeorge syndrome, in which TOF is often a factor. Additionally, single-gene defects may also be associated with specific structural CHD. For example, supravalvular stenosis is associated with Williams syndrome, for which a genetic test is available.

Cardiovascular genetic and molecular researchers have used genetic testing for cardiac channelopathies, such as LQTS and BrS, for the past decade, and these have recently become available commercially. In May of 2004, the first commercial test was released by Genaissance Pharmaceuticals [75]. The test, known by the name FAMILION, provides a comprehensive mutational analysis of the five cardiac channel genes implicated in LQTS or a SCN5A-targeted test [75]. Insurance providers are increasing their coverage of genetic testing and researchers have concluded that the test is cost effective in familial LQTS as opposed to no testing, at an estimated cost of $2500 dollars per year of life saved [76].

Sensitivity and specificity of LQTS commercial testing is reportedly high. Mutations are found in 50% to 75% of LQTS cases and 15% to 30% of BrS cases [74]. Efforts continue to improve the quality of testing. In 2006 Tester and colleagues [77] identified allelic dropout as a mechanism for obtaining false-negative results in patients who had LQTS and recommended that particular attention be paid to regions susceptible to allele dropout. Currently 1211 diseases are tested for by laboratories certified by the Clinical Laboratory Improvement Amendment (CLIA) to do clinical testing. There are an additional 288 diseases tested for within the framework of research studies. The University of Washington provides a Web site sponsored by the National Institutes of Health (www.genetests.org) [78]. This site provides frequently updated information regarding genetic testing and a laboratory directory of clinics that offer molecular genetic testing, specialized cytogenetic testing, and biochemical testing for inherited disorders in the United States and worldwide.

In summary, despite the enormous advances made in the field of molecular genetics, new knowledge is being gained every day. Nurses caring for children or adults who have CHD and their families must constantly educate themselves by keeping abreast of current information. By being knowledgeable, cardiovascular nurses can provide the most current and up-to-date care for their patients who have heritable cardiac conditions.

References

[1] Webb GD, Smallhorn JF, Therrien J, et al. Congenital heart disease. In: Zipes DP, Libby P, Bonow RO, et al, editors. Braunwald's heart disease: a textbook of cardiovascular medicine. 2nd edition. Philadelphia: Elsevier Saunders; 2005. p. 1489–552.

[2] Hoffman JI, Kaplan S. The incidence of congenital heart disease. J Am Coll Cardiol 2002;39:1890–900.

[3] Gill HK, Splitt M, Sharland GK, et al. Patterns of recurrence of congenital heart disease. An analysis of 6,640 consecutive pregnancies evaluated by detailed fetal echocardiography. J Am Coll Cardiol 2003;42(5):923–9.

[4] Jenkins KJ, Correa A, Feinstein JA, et al. Noninherited risk factors and congenital cardiovascular defects: current knowledge. Circulation 2007;115: 2995–3014.

[5] Pierpont ME, Basson CT, Benson DW, et al. Genetic basis for congenital heart defects: current knowledge. Circulation 2007;115:3015–38.

[6] Rome JJ, Kruetzer J. Pediatric interventional catheterization: reasonable expectations and outcomes. Pediatr Clin North Am 2004;51(12):1589–610.

[7] Zetterqvist P. Multiple occurrence of atrial septal defect in a family. Acta Paediatr 1960;49:741–7.

[8] Zuckerman HS, Zuckerman GH, Mammen RE, et al. Atrial septal defect: familial occurrence in four generations of one family. Am J Cardiol 1962; 9:515–20.

[9] Benson DW, Sharkey A, Fatkin D, et al. Reduced penetrance, variable expressivity, and genetic heterogeneity of familial atrial septal defects. Circulation 1998;97:2043–8.

[10] Online mendelian inheritance in man. Available at: www.ncbi.nlm.nih.gov/omim/. Accessed October 22, 2007.

[11] Digilio MC, Marino B, Cicini MP, et al. Risk of congenital heart defects in relatives of patients with atrioventricular canal. Am J Dis Child 1993;147: 1295–7.

[12] Sheffield VC, Pierpont ME, Nishimura D, et al. Identification of a complex congenital heart defect susceptibility locus using DNA pooling and shared segment analysis. Hum Mol Genet 1997;6:117–21.

[13] Eisenberg R, Young D, Jacobson B, et al. Familial supravalvular aortic stenosis. Am J Dis Child 1964; 108:341–7.

[14] Lewis AJ, Ongley PA, Kincaid OW, et al. Supravalvular aortic stenosis. Report of a family with peculiar somatic features and normal intelligence. Dis Chest 1969;55:372–9.

[15] Curran ME, Atkinson DL, Ewart AK, et al. The elastin gene is disrupted by a translocation associated with supravalvular aortic stenosis. Cell 1993; 73:159–68.

[16] Ewart AK, Morris CA, Ensing GJ, et al. A human vascular disorder, supravalvular aortic stenosis, maps to chromosome 7. Proc Natl Acad Sci U S A 1993;90:3226–30.

[17] Kumar A, Olson TM, Thibodeau SN, et al. Confirmation of linkage of supravalvular aortic stenosis to the elastin gene on chromosome 7q. Am J Cardiol 1994;74:1281–3.

[18] Cripe L, Andelfinger G, Martin LJ, et al. Bicuspid aortic valve is heritable. J Am Coll Cardiol 2004; 44:138–42.

[19] Gough JH. Coarctation of the aorta in father and son. Br J Radiol 1961;34:670–4.

[20] Beekman RH, Robinow M. Coarctation of the aorta inherited as an autosomal dominant trait. Am J Cardiol 1985;56:818–9.

[21] Loffredo CA, Chokkalingam A, Sill AM, et al. Prevalence of congenital cardiovascular malformations among relatives of infants with hypoplastic left heart, coarctation of the aorta, and d-transposition of the great arteries. Am J Med Genet A 2004;124:225–30.

[22] Wessels MW, Berger RM, Frohn-Mulder IME, et al. Autosomal dominant inheritance of left ventricular outflow tract obstruction. Am J Med Genet A 2005;134:171–9.

[23] McBride KL, Pignatelli R, Lewin M, et al. Inheritance analysis of congenital left ventricular outflow tract obstruction malformations: segregation, multiplex relative risk, and heritability. Am J Med Genet A 2005;134:180–6.

[24] Digilio MC, Marino B, Giannotti A, et al. Recurrence risk figures for isolated tetralogy of Fallot after screening for 22q11 microdeletion. J Med Genet 1997;34:188–90.

[25] Hirt-Armon K, Pober BR, Holmes LB. Type III tracheal agenesis with familial tetralogy of Fallot and absent pulmonary valve syndrome. Am J Med Genet 1996;65:266–8.

[26] Benson DW, Silberbach GM, Kavanaugh-McHugh A, et al. Mutations in the cardiac transcription factor NKX2.5 affect diverse cardiac developmental pathways. J Clin Invest 1999;104:1567–73.

[27] Eldadah ZA, Hamosh A, Biery NJ, et al. Familial tetralogy of Fallot caused by mutation in the jagged1 gene. Hum Molec Genet 2001;10:163–9.

[28] Goldmuntz E, Geiger E, Benson DW. NKX2.5 mutations in patients with tetralogy of Fallot. Circulation 2001;104:2565–8.

[29] Becker TA, Van Amber R, Moller JH, et al. Occurrence of cardiac malformations in relatives of children with transposition of the great arteries. Am J Med Genet 1996;66:28–32.

[30] Goldmuntz E, Bamford R, Karkera JD, et al. CFC1 mutations in patients with transposition of the great arteries and double-outlet right ventricle. Am J Hum Genet 2002;70:776–80.

[31] Muncke N, Jung C, Rüdiger H, et al. Missense mutations and gene interruption in PROSIT240, a novel TRAP240-like gene, in patients with congenital heart defect (transposition of the great arteries). Circulation 2003;108:2843–50.

[32] Pierpont MEM, Gobel JW, Moller JH, et al. Cardiac malformations in relatives of children with truncus arteriosus or interruption of the aortic arch. Am J Cardiol 1988;61:423–7.

[33] Rein AJ, Dollberg S, Gale R. Genetics of conotruncal malformations: review of the literature and report of a consanguineous kindred with various conotruncal malformations. Am J Med Genet 1990; 36:353–5.

[34] Rein AJJT, Sheffer R. Genetics of conotruncal malformations: further evidence of autosomal recessive inheritance [letter]. Am J Med Genet 1994;50: 302–3.

[35] Matsuoka R, Kimura M, Scambler PJ, et al. Molecular and clinical study of 183 patients with conotruncal anomaly face syndrome. Hum Genet 1998;103: 70–80.

[36] Matsuok R, Takao A, Kimura M, et al. Confirmation that the conotruncal anomaly face syndrome is associated with a deletion within 22q11.2. Am J Med Genet 1994;53:285–9.

[37] Yagi H, Furutani Y, Hamada H, et al. Role of TBX1 in human del22q11.2 syndrome. Lancet 2003;362: 1366–73.

[38] Shokeir MH. Hypoplastic left heart syndrome: an autosomal recessive disorder. Clin Genet 1971;2: 7–14.

[39] Holmes LB, Rose V, Child AH, et al. Commentary on the inheritance of the hypoplastic left heart syndrome. Birth Defects Orig Artic Ser 1974;X: 228–30.

[40] Brownell LG, Shokeir MH. Inheritance of hypoplastic left heart syndrome (HLHS): further observations. Clin Genet 1976;9:245–9.

[41] Hinton RB Jr, Martin LJ, Tabangin ME, et al. Hypoplastic left heart is heritable. J Am Coll Cardiol 2007;50:1590–5.

[42] Noonan JA, Ehmke DA. Associated noncardiac malformations in children with congenital heart disease. J Pediatr 1975;63:468–70.

[43] Greenwood RD, Rosenthal A, Paris L, et al. Extracardiac abnormalities in infants with congenital heart disease. Pediatrics 1975;55:485–92.

[44] Schnizel AP. Catalogue of unbalanced chromosome aberrations in man. New York: Walter de Gruyter; 1984.

[45] Towbin JA, Greenberg FG. Genetic syndromes and clinical molecular genetics. In: Garson A Jr, Bricker JT, Fisher DJ, et al, editors. The science and practice of pediatric cardiology. 2nd edition. Baltimore (MD): Williams and Wilkins; 1998. p. 2627–99.

[46] Rehder H. Pathology of trisomy 21 with particular reference to persistent common atrioventricular canal of the heart. In: Bugio GR, editor. Trisomy 21. New York: Springer-Verlag; 1981. p. 57–73.

[47] Allanson JE. Noonan syndrome. J Med Genet 1987; 24:9–13.

[48] Burch M, Sharland M, Shinebourne E, et al. Cardiologic abnormalities in Noonan syndrome: phenotypic diagnosis and electrocardiographic assessment of 118 patients. J Am Coll Cardiol 1993;22:1189–92.

[49] DiGeorge AM. Discussions on the new concept of the cellular basis of immunity. Journal of Pediatrics 1965;67:907–8.

[50] Pierpont ME, Moller JM. The genetics of cardiovascular disease. Hingham (MA): Martinus Nijhoff; 1985.

[51] Keppen LD, Fasules JW, Burks AW, et al. Confirmation of autosomal dominant transmission of the DiGeorge malformation complex. J Pediatr 1988; 113:506–8.

[52] Goldmuntz E. DiGeorge syndrome: new insights. Clin Perinatol 2005;32:963–78.

[53] Jervell A, Lange-Nielsen F. Congenital deaf-mutism, functional heart disease with prolongation of the QT and sudden death. Am Heart J 1957;54: 59–68.

[54] Tomasselli GF. A failure to adapt: ankyrins in congenital and acquired arrhythmias. Circulation 2007;115:428–9.

[55] Schwertz DW, Aouizerat BE, Wung SF. Genetic and environmental basis of cardiac disease. In: Moser DK, Riegel B, editors. Cardiac nursing. A companion to Braunwald's heart disease. St. Louis (MO): Saunders Elsevier; 2008. p. 171–87.

[56] Romano C, Gemme G, Pongiglione R. Rare cardiac arrhythmias of the pediatric age. I. Repetitive paroxysmal tachycardia. Minerva Pediatr 1963;15: 1155–64. Italian.

[57] Ward OC. A new familial cardiac syndrome in children. J Ir Med Assoc 1964;54:103–6.

[58] Neyroud N, Tesson F, Denjoy I, et al. A novel mutation in the potassium channel gene KVLQT1 causes the Jervell and Lange-Nielsen cardioauditory syndrome. Nat Genet 1997;15:186–9.

[59] Keating M, Dunn C, Atkinson D, et al. Consistent linkage of the long-QT syndrome to the Harvey Ras-1 locus on chromosome 11. Am J Hum Genet 1991;49:1335–9.

[60] Tester DJ, Will ML, Ackerman MJ. Mutation detection in congenital long QT syndrome: cardiac channel gene screen using PCR, dHPLC, and direct DNA sequencing. Methods Mol Med 2006;128: 181–207, 64.

[61] Priori SG, Napolitano C, Schwartz PJ. Genetics of cardiac arrhythmias. In: Zipes DP, Libby P, Bonow RO, et al, editors. Braunwald's heart disease. A textbook of cardiovascular medicine. 7th edition. Philadelphia: Elsevier Saunders; 2005. p. 689–95.

[62] Locati EH, Zareba W, Moss AJ, et al. Age- and sex-related differences in clinical manifestations in patients with congenital long-QT syndrome. Circulation 1998;97:2237–44.

[63] Schwartz PJ, Priori SG, Spazzolini C, et al. Genotype-phenotype correlation in the long-QT syndrome. Gene-specific triggers for life-threatening arrhythmias. Circulation 2001;103:89–95.

[64] Martini B, Nava A, Thiene G, et al. Ventricular fibrillation without apparent heart disease: description of six cases. Am Heart J 1989;118:1203–9.

[65] Brugada P, Brugada J. Right bundle branch block, persistent ST segment elevation and sudden cardiac death: a distinct clinical and electrocardiographic syndrome: a multicenter report. J Am Coll Cardiol 1992;20:1391–6.

[66] Rook MB, Alshinawi CB, Groenewegen WA, et al. Human SCN5A gene mutations alter cardiac sodium channel kinetics and are associated with the Brugada syndrome. Cardiovasc Res 1999;44: 507–17.

[67] Priori SG, Napolitano C, Gasparini M, et al. Natural history of Brugada syndrome: insights for risk stratification and management. Circulation 2002; 105:1342–7.

[68] Weiss R, Barmada MM, Nguyen T, et al. Clinical and molecular heterogeneity in the Brugada syndrome: a novel gene locus on chromosome 3. Circulation 2002;105:707–13.

[69] Coumel P, Fidelle J, Lucet V, et al. Catecholaminergic-induced severe ventricular arrhythmias with Adams-Stokes syndrome in children: report of four cases. British Heart Journal 1978;40:28–37.

[70] Leenhardt A, Lucet V, Denjoy I, et al. Catecholaminergic polymorphic ventricular tachycardia in children: a 7-year follow-up of 21 patients. Circulation 1995;91:1512–9.

[71] Priori SG, Napolitano C, Tiso N, et al. Mutations in the cardiac ryanodine receptor gene (hRyR2) underlie catecholaminergic polymorphic ventricular tachycardia. Circulation 2000;102:r49–53.

[72] Laitinen PJ, Brown KM, Piippo K, et al. Mutations of the cardiac ryanodine receptor (RyR2) gene in familial polymorphic ventricular tachycardia. Circulation 2001;103:485–90.

[73] Lahat H, Pras E, Olender T, et al. A missense mutation in a highly conserved region of CASQ2 is associated with autosomal recessive catecholamine-induced polymorphic ventricular tachycardia in Bedouin families from Israel. Am J Hum Genet 2001;69:1378–84.

[74] Benson DW, Wang DW, Dyment M, et al. Congenital sick sinus syndrome caused by recessive mutations in the cardiac sodium channel gene (SCN5A). J Clin Invest 2003;112:1019–28.

[75] Tester DJ, Ackerman MJ. Genetic testing for cardiac channelopathies: ten questions regarding clinical considerations for heart rhythm allied professionals. Heart Rhythm 2005;2:675–7.

[76] Phillips KA, Ackerman MJ, Sakowski J, et al. Cost-effectiveness analysis of genetic testing for familial long QT syndrome in symptomatic index cases. Heart Rhythm 2005;2:1294–300.

[77] Tester DJ, Cronk LB, Carr JL, et al. Allelic dropout in long QT syndrome genetic testing: a possible mechanism underlying false-negative results. Heart Rhythm 2006;3:815–21.

[78] Gene Tests. University of Seattle at Washington. Retrieved from December 2, 2007. Available at: http://www.genetests.org/. Accessed December 6, 2007.

CRITICAL CARE
NURSING CLINICS
OF NORTH AMERICA

Crit Care Nurs Clin N Am 20 (2008) 171–189

Genetic Influences in Common Respiratory Disorders

M. Linda Workman, PhD, RN, FAAN[a],*,
Chris Winkelman, RN, PhD, CCRN, ACNP[b]

[a]College of Nursing, University of Cincinnati, Cincinnati, OH, USA
[b]Frances Payne Bolton School of Nursing, Case Western Reserve University, 10900 Euclid Avenue,
Cleveland, OH 44106-4904, USA

Overview

The expression of many common respiratory disorders of adults and children is the result of a gene–environment interaction in which the susceptibility to the development of the problem has a genetic basis and the environment influences its age at onset, variability, severity, and, to some extent, its pathologic progression. With any of these disorders, the genetic influences and environmental influences are not equal and are not yet completely understood. For some problems, such as cystic fibrosis, the genetic influence is far greater than the environmental influence (Fig. 1). For other problems, such as pulmonary infection and problems associated with pulmonary trauma, the environmental influence is greater than the genetic influence, although the genetic influence is still present and seems to affect the individual's physiologic responses and the consequences of the environmental insult.

Even those pulmonary problems that are largely environmental issues, such as pneumonia and tuberculosis that require environmental exposure to the infectious organisms for infection development, respond to genetic influences. Susceptibility to the development of infection in the presence of any given microorganism is not equal among humans. Evidence of variable susceptibility to infection is demonstrated by infectious epidemics during past centuries in which some individuals became ill and succumbed to the disease, some became ill and recovered from the disease, and others equally exposed escaped unscathed even when all other members of a household succumbed to the infection. Genetic variation among families and individuals, especially among factors regulating immunity and inflammatory responses, influences susceptibility to infection [1].

Susceptibility and resistance

Some genetic variants in a gene or genes can lead to an increased susceptibility for a specific disease or disorder. For example, having one mutated allele in the BRCA1 gene increases a woman's risk for breast cancer development from an overall 12% lifetime risk to a lifetime risk of 60% to 80%. This same mutation increases the lifetime risk for ovarian cancer development from about 1.5% to a risk of 60% to 80%. Such gene mutations that are known to greatly increase risk are called susceptibility genes. Although the presence of a susceptibility gene increases the risk for disease, the risk seldom is 100%. Whether or not this increased genetic risk is ever expressed is partly determined by the presence of other genetic variations that seem to provide some protective influence.

Numerous known gene variants exist as susceptibility genes, such as those that are associated with the development of Huntington disease, sickle cell disease, colorectal cancer, familial hypercholesterolemia, hereditary hemochromatosis, long QT syndrome, and achondroplasia, to name only a few [2]. These susceptibility genes

* Corresponding author. 8727 Tanagerwoods Drive, Cincinnati, OH 45249.

E-mail address: mlindaworkman@gmail.com (M.L. Workman).

Genetic Influence   **Environmental Influence**

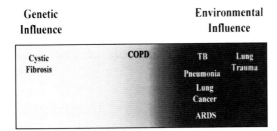

Fig. 1. Expression of selected complex pulmonary problems as a result of the interaction between genetic and environmental influences.

result in single-gene–type expression patterns that may be autosomal dominant, autosomal recessive, or sex-linked recessive. It is also believed that many more susceptibility variations may exist within more than one gene, requiring a "group effect" to increase specific health problem susceptibility. These variations are most likely to occur in the genes coding for proteins that regulate enzyme activity, inflammation and immune responses, and metabolism.

Genes that can provide protection against the development or expression of a specific disease are called resistance genes or modifier genes. Currently, much more is known about susceptibility genes than is known about resistance genes.

For many complex disorders that have a strong genetic component, the expression of the disorder represents an imbalance between those susceptibility genes that promote expression and those resistance genes that protect against expression. Fig. 2 demonstrates the influence of genetic susceptibility on the expression of a health problem and Fig. 3 demonstrates the theoretic influence of genetic resistance on the expression of a health problem.

Some autosomal recessive gene variations seem to have been acquired through evolution to increase individual resistance to a particular health problem and are said to confer a selection advantage or a survival advantage to the carrying individual over individuals who do not have the "abnormal" variation. Such variations are overall beneficial in the heterozygous state, but may be catastrophic in the homozygous state.

One such gene variation is the single nucleotide substitution in the gene coding for the β-chain of hemoglobin. Individuals who are heterozygous (have the mutation in only one gene allele) for this variation have sickle cell trait, which rarely causes clinical problems but confers resistance to

malaria. Those individuals who are homozygous (have the mutation in both gene alleles) for the mutation have sickle cell disease, which is a serious life-limiting disorder. Considering that the heterozygous state is present in about 1 out of 12 to 1 out of 15 African Americans and the homozygous state is present in about 1 out of 400 African Americans [2], it is easy to see that historically many more individuals were able to benefit from the malarial protection of the heterozygous state than were harmed by the homozygous state.

Another group of autosomal recessive gene variations with a widespread presence in certain racial and ethnic populations and theorized to confer a survival advantage occurs in the cystic fibrosis gene (CTFR). The high frequency of the heterozygous state among whites from Northern and Western Europe suggested a possible advantage. Recent evidence indicates that individuals who are heterozygous for specific common CFTR mutations seem to be resistant to typhoid and to cholera toxin when exposed to these disease-causing microorganisms [3]. This genetic disorder is discussed in more detail later in this article.

Environmental influences

Genetic influences (nature) for or against health problem expression also are affected by environmental (nurturing) conditions. For example, a person who has increased genetic susceptibility to tuberculosis and decreased genetic resistance to the disease may never develop the disease because of a lack of environmental exposure to the causative organism. In addition to the external environmental factor, the environment also includes how the person nurtures or cares for his or her personal or internal environment. Such factors include level of nutrition, intact barriers, and lack of physical or psychologic stressors.

One common example of a disorder with increased genetic susceptibility is type 2 diabetes mellitus. Gestational diabetes during pregnancy confirmed by abnormal glucose tolerance is highly predictive of the later development of type 2 diabetes mellitus. A person who knows this risk may choose to alter her internal environment to increase environmental resistance to this disease. Such alterations include maintaining an appropriate body weight, limiting intake of carbohydrates and fats, and engaging in a consistent program of aerobic exercise. These personal environment alterations have been shown to delay the onset

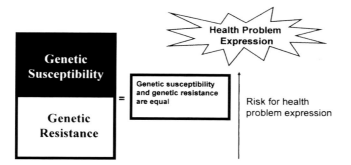

Susceptibility and resistance factors are balanced.
No increased genetic risk

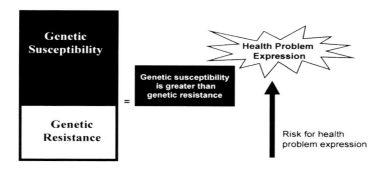

Genetic susceptibility is greater than normal with only a normal
level of genetic resistance. Conditions are unbalanced, resulting
in an increased genetic risk.

Fig. 2. Influences of genetic susceptibility in health problem expression.

of the disorder by decades and even prevent its expression altogether in some cases. It therefore may be possible to "beat your genes" in the positive direction even when a known genetic susceptibility or predisposition exists.

Common complex disorders often represent a gene–environment interaction for development. When genetic susceptibility and genetic resistance are balanced with environmental susceptibility and environmental resistance, personal risk for health problem expression does not increase (Fig. 4). In addition, when environmental causes or mediators for a genetic health problem are known, environmental manipulation can be used to counter increased genetic susceptibility or decreased genetic resistance (Fig. 5). For example, the presence of specific mutations in both gene alleles for α_1-antitrypsin (AAT) greatly increases the risk for the expression of emphysema at an early age among cigarette smokers. The risk is made worse if the individual also has a mutation in an enzyme metabolism gene that clears the toxins

present in inhaled cigarette smoke from the body. These two conditions thus represent greatly increased genetic susceptibility and decreased genetic resistance. Manipulation of the environment by not smoking and by avoiding other types of particulate matter inhalation moderates the genetic risks by reducing or eliminating the environmental risk. This type of theoretic model works well when the genetic and the environmental influences regarding specific health problem expression are known; unfortunately, the gene–environment interactions for many common and complex health problems have not yet been elucidated.

Noninfectious disorders

Cystic fibrosis

Early history

Cystic fibrosis (CF) is a classic model of genetic susceptibility. It is a genetic disorder with an autosomal recessive pattern of inheritance that

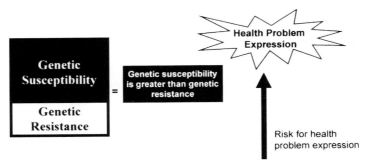

Genetic susceptibility is normal with less than normal genetic resistance.
Conditions are unbalanced resulting in an increased genetic risk.

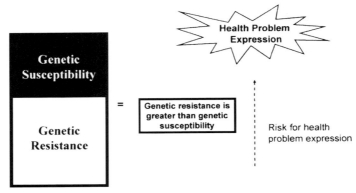

Genetic susceptibility normal with greater than normal genetic resistance.
Genetic risk is NOT increased.

Fig. 3. Influences of genetic resistance in health problem expression.

affects many organs and has the potential to lethally impair pulmonary function. What is suspected to be the most severe form of the disorder was first described centuries ago as the result of "bewitched" infants [4]. These babies, who tasted salty when kissed, were considered bewitched and doomed to an early death from poor nutrition, diarrhea, and difficulty breathing. In the twentieth century, the name "cystic fibromatosis with bronchiectasis" was first used in association with the condition, although the most pressing clinical issue at that time was believed to be pancreatic dysfunction. By 1938, a more comprehensive description of the clinical manifestations of the disorder was presented [5], along with documentation of the universal presence of thick sticky mucus [4]. In the mid 1940s, enough information from kinship studies had been gathered to establish that CF seemed to follow an autosomal recessive inheritance pattern and most likely was the result of a mutation in a single gene [6].

Testing for diagnosis of CF had its roots in 1953 when di Sant'agnese and colleagues [7] noted that the sweat of CF patients had excessively high levels of sodium chloride. By 1958 the sweat chloride test was developed and remains a diagnostic tool for CF still in use today [4]. Just how this salty sweat could possibly be related to cysts, fibrosis, and the large quantity of mucus that formed plugs in many organs could not be explained.

The combination of the clinical manifestations coupled with a positive sweat chloride test provided an accurate diagnosis of CF for the homozygous individual who actually expressed the disease. The heterozygous carrier, however, could not be identified using these means.

Clinical picture

The comprehensive clinical picture of this disorder showed three primary tissue problems that seemed to be epithelial in nature. The

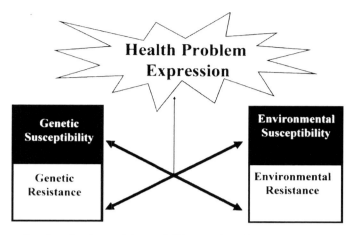

Genetic and environmental susceptibilities are balanced by environmental and genetic resistance – no overall increased risk for health problem expression.

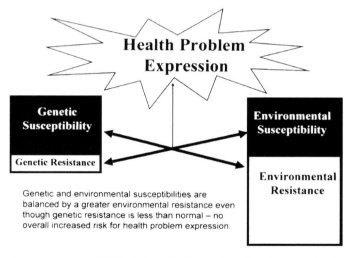

Genetic and environmental susceptibilities are balanced by a greater environmental resistance even though genetic resistance is less than normal – no overall increased risk for health problem expression.

Fig. 4. Genetic and environmental susceptibilities balanced with genetic and environmental resistance to maintain a low risk for health problem expression.

epithelial tissues produce a thick, sticky mucus that causes problems in the lungs, exocrine pancreas (non-hormone-secreting), liver, salivary glands, and testes. Essentially, the mucus plugs up glands in these organs, causing glandular atrophy and organ dysfunction.

The pulmonary problems of CF result from the constant presence of thick, sticky mucus and are the most serious complications of the disease. The mucus narrows airways, reducing airflow. The constant presence of mucus results in chronic lower respiratory bacterial infections with chronic bronchitis, bronchiectasis, increased alveolar compliance, and lung abscesses. Changes occur

in the bronchiole over time, including bronchiole distension along with hyperplasia and hypertrophy of mucus-producing cells. Pulmonary complications of CF are common and include pneumothorax, arterial erosion and hemorrhage, antibiotic-resistant infection, and respiratory failure [2].

Pancreatic problems from mucus changes lead to plugging of the exocrine ducts with resulting gland atrophy and progressive fibrotic cyst formation. The endocrine function of the CF pancreas is largely unaffected. These atrophic and fibrotic changes cause a reduced to eventually absent production of the digestive enzymes lipase,

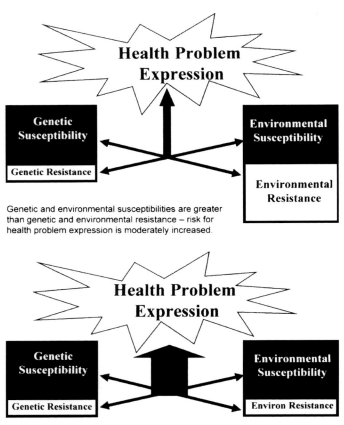

Genetic and environmental susceptibilities are greater than genetic and environmental resistance – risk for health problem expression is moderately increased.

Genetic and environmental susceptibilities overwhelm genetic and environmental resistance – risk for health problem expression is greatly increased.

Fig. 5. Genetic and environmental susceptibilities not balanced with genetic and environmental resistance, leading to varying degrees of increased risk for health problem expression.

trypsin, and chymotrypsin, which are needed for fat and protein nutrient digestion. Inadequate levels of these enzymes leads to malnutrition, smaller stature, steatorrhea, and deficiency of fat-soluble vitamins. In about 10% of patients who have CF, the pancreatic pathology is present in the prenatal period and these infants are born with an intestinal obstruction created by a meconium ileus, a condition termed "mucoviscidosis" [8]. These primary nonpulmonary problems cause a multitude of secondary problems.

Other digestive organs also are affected by CF. The liver and gall bladder are damaged by mucus deposits and concretions although the gall bladder damage may not be clinically detectable for the first 3 decades of life. The liver becomes cirrhotic over time. Although liver failure is a late development, children often have focal areas of ductal dilation and cirrhosis from granular mucus plugs. Salivary gland ducts are often dilated and the composition of saliva is atypical. The origin of the salivary changes is not precisely known and may be related to the disease itself or to the pharmacologic management of CF.

Male infertility is associated with CF, although this is a more recent finding because many children who had the most severe form of CF did not live to reach reproductive functional capacity. Most adult males who have CF have no sperm present in the seminal fluid. The pathologic issue is an absence of the vas deferens, termed agenesis of the vas deferens (VF) [9]. The function of the VF is to transport spermatozoa from testicular storage sites to the penile urethra. Without VF development, the individual produces spermatozoa that never enter the ejaculated fluid.

One confusing issue noted with the clinical presentation of CF was its variability in severity and in organ involvement. Usually within a family, the clinical course was consistent for the individuals diagnosed with the disease. Greater variation in severity and age of symptom onset was noted in different families. In one family, for example, affected individuals were diagnosed during infancy and progressed with relative rapidity to end-stage pulmonary failure in only a few years. In other families, the symptoms were not as obvious and individuals were not diagnosed until later childhood or adolescence. A few individuals were not diagnosed until adulthood and may have only expressed pancreatic manifestations or pulmonary manifestations.

Diagnostic progress

During the 1970s, gel electrophoresis of plasma proteins gained popularity as a research and clinical tool. Considering the implications of mutation in a single gene as the basis for CF, it seemed logical that the homozygous condition would produce an abnormal electrophoretic pattern that could be used to distinguish those who had CF (homozygotes) from those who were carriers (heterozygotes) and from those who did not have a copy of the abnormal gene allele. This process was attempted and successful to a degree. Even though the actual protein had yet to be identified, within a family unit affected individuals, carriers, and completely unaffected individuals could be identified. Usually, the blood of the person who had CF would show a unique protein band in a specific position on the gel. Blood from family members who were carriers of the abnormal gene allele, but who did not have CF, showed a smaller but distinct protein band in the same position as the affected individual. Family members whose blood did not show any protein band at the same position were considered to be neither affected nor carriers. What was puzzling was that the electrophoretic protein band patterns were not the same for all families who had members who had CF. Each family thus needed to have electrophoresis of the person who had CF performed first to be able to extrapolate accurately the carrier versus the noncarrier status of other family members.

In 1985 the gene responsible for CF was localized to chromosome 7 [10]. By 1989 the gene locus was mapped precisely to 7q31 [11]. This gene, cystic fibrosis transmembrane conductance regulator (CFTR), has more than one function. The main function is that of a chloride channel, regulating chloride and bicarbonate transport [12]. It also is involved with controlling or regulating other transport pathways.

During the intervening years from mapping and sequencing the gene, more has come to light regarding the puzzles of variation in manifestations and variation in the gel electrophoresis of the protein coded by the gene. The gene and its product are complex. Different regions of the gene code for different parts of the protein that have varying roles in development and physiologic function. The epithelial tissues are most affected by the abnormal protein and the exact link between electrolyte transport and mucus abnormalities is not completely known, although issues of cellular nutrition and energy production or use have been raised [12].

Currently, more than 1000 different mutations in this gene have been identified and are believed to account for much of the variance in severity, age of symptom onset, and differences in organ involvement [2,13]. Although there are so many mutations, some are more common than others, with the F508 being the most common and its consequences the most severe [14]. Although the entire human spectrum of possible CFTR mutations is not yet known, most of the known mutations do not prevent the synthesis of this protein. Rather, the mutations slightly change the protein sequence and structure to the extent that, depending on which mutation is present, the protein still functions but to different levels of efficiency. The genotype of the problem (which mutation is present) can now better be correlated to the specific phenotype (clinical manifestations) expressed by the person who has CF [13].

Clinical implications

Cystic fibrosis carrier status is most prevalent in whites from northern and western Europe with an estimated frequency of 1 in 20. Approximately 1 out of every 2500 births of individuals in this ethnic group is homozygous and expresses the disease [2]. Although more prevalent in whites, the disorder is expressed in individuals of all races but to a much lesser extent. With the discovery of true CF existing in more mild forms that may go undiagnosed until middle adulthood, it seems that the prevalence is considerably higher than previously calculated.

Once considered exclusively a childhood disorder, people who have severe forms of CF are living longer and are undergoing aggressive therapies, such as lung transplantation, in acute care settings. With improvement in specific testing, people who have health problems who were not known to have CF previously may be identified so that therapies can be tailored for greater efficacy. In critical care settings, patients who have what seem to be acute pulmonary problems who do not respond as expected to proven therapy may, in actuality, have some undiagnosed form of CF that unfavorably influences the clinical course of a superimposed pulmonary problem [15,16]. Although testing of such individuals is not currently feasible, the future of individualized health problem management may be possible when the multitude of CFTR genotypes is known and techniques, such as microarray mutation analysis, become common and affordable. In addition, the day of gene therapy for cystic fibrosis is coming closer.

Chronic obstructive pulmonary disease

Disease overview

Chronic obstructive pulmonary disease (COPD) is an acquired progressive respiratory disorder that is usually expressed as a combination of emphysema and chronic bronchitis with significant symptoms manifesting in the sixth and seventh decades of life [17]. Each condition has its own pathophysiologic process and any individual who has COPD may show a predominance of either disorder. The major risk factor for both conditions is cigarette smoking, which would seem to place COPD closer toward the environmental side of the gene–environment interaction continuum (see Fig. 1). COPD is not an equal opportunity disease, however, considering two known facts. First, only about 15% of smokers develop clinically relevant manifestations [18]; second, families have been identified in which the disease presents at a far earlier than expected average age. Both facts suggest the existence of genetic factors influencing environmental susceptibility.

In the healthy lung, protein-degrading enzymes called proteases are present to destroy and eliminate protein-based particulate matter and microorganisms inhaled during ventilation or trapped in the microvasculature of the lungs as a result of translocation from other body sites during circulation. These proteases include elastase and trypsin, among others. In addition, macrophages and neutrophils, along with their associated proteolytic enzymes, contact the lungs many times per second during normal circulation [19]. The action of the proteases is controlled by other protease-inhibiting enzymes, called protease inhibitors or PIs, to prevent enzyme damage to those proteins forming the anatomic structures of the lungs. The most common PI is α_1-antitrypsin (AAT), which is synthesized in the liver and in macrophages and neutrophils [19]. Liver-synthesized AAT is released into the blood where it circulates to the lungs to exert its protease-inhibiting action. The healthy lung thus has well-regulated processes to limit or prevent indiscriminate protein destruction while ensuring efficient removal of unwanted protein. Chronic exposure to cigarette smoke, coal dust, or other particulate matter increases gene transcription and induces greater production of proteases to inactivate or eliminate these external protein-based inhalation irritants. When the countering activity or amounts of PIs increase proportionately to balance the increased amounts of proteases, only the particulate matter is affected and normal pulmonary structures remain undamaged.

Pathophysiology

Emphysema is the result of loss of alveolar elasticity (recoil) resulting in pathologically increased pulmonary compliance, lung hyperinflation, and increased residual volume preventing effective gas exchange at the alveolar–capillary interface. The cause of emphysema is believed to be an imbalance in which protease activity is greater than the balancing PI activity, especially AAT activity [17,19]. Either protease production is so greatly increased that these enzymes escape the controlling capacity of PIs, or the PIs are present in suboptimal concentrations and cannot increase to balance the presence of the proteases. Protease activity thus is not confined to the degradation of unwanted proteins and now damages elastin, pulmonary connective tissue, and the alveoli. As result, the alveoli are damaged and lose elasticity followed by overstretching and enlargement into air-filled spaces called bullae. The smaller bronchioles then collapse, greatly increasing the work of breathing.

Bronchitis is an inflammation of the bronchi and bronchioles caused by continuous exposure to infectious or noninfectious irritants, especially tobacco smoke. The irritant produces an inflammatory response resulting in vasodilation, congestion, mucosal edema, and bronchospasm. Unlike emphysema, bronchitis affects the airways rather than the alveoli [17].

Chronic inflammation results in mucus gland hypertrophy and hyperplasia, which produce large amounts of thick mucus. The bronchial walls thicken and impair airflow, which together with production of excessive mucus hinders airflow and increases the risk for secondary infections.

Clinical picture

The major clinical manifestation of clinically recognizable COPD is dyspnea. The hyperinflated lung flattens the diaphragm, weakening the effect of this major muscle of respiration. As a result, the person who has emphysema needs to use accessory muscles in the neck, chest wall, and abdomen to inhale and exhale. This increased effort increases the need for oxygen and metabolic nutrients, making the patient work harder and experience an air-hunger sensation. The narrowed airways lead to wheezing and inhalation usually starts before exhalation is completed, resulting in dyspnea with an uncoordinated pattern of breathing.

In advanced disease, the person is usually thin, with a large, rounded thorax that appears out of proportion to the rest of the body's size. Ribs are widely spaced and the sternocleidomastoid muscles are well developed. Nail beds are cyanotic with clubbing of the fingers. The face and oral mucus membranes are dusky. Respirations are shallow and rapid, with the person unable to complete a sentence without pausing for breath. Mucus and sputum production are increased and lower respiratory infections are common.

Gas exchange is affected by the increased work of breathing and the loss of alveolar tissue. Although some alveoli enlarge, the curves of alveolar walls decrease and there is less surface area available for gas exchange. The typical arterial blood gas (ABG) changes associated with the advanced COPD are low pH, high $Paco_2$, low Pao_2, and high bicarbonate levels. The acidosis is not as severe as it could be, given the derangement of poor oxygen diffusion and excess carbon dioxide retention, as a result of renal compensation with increased reabsorption of bicarbonate and increased excretion of urinary hydrogen ions.

Genetic features

Clustering of COPD among smoking family members in the third and fourth decades of life first triggered an interest in exploring additional risk factors for the disorder. In the 1960s the finding of low serum levels of AAT among patients who had early-onset disease set the stage for better characterization of genetic involvement [20–23]. One issue that suggested more than one genetic mutation was the variance in clinical manifestations among individuals who had early-age onset. Some patients had only pulmonary involvement, some had pulmonary and liver involvement, and a very few others expressed only liver involvement. The liver disease associated with deficiency of AAT was characterized by the presence of intracellular deposits that formed inclusion bodies and damaged hepatocytes. Progression of deposit formation led to eventual liver cirrhosis. Other associated diseases or manifestations that occasionally accompanied AAT deficiency included arterial aneurysm, rheumatoid arthritis, renal disease, and certain cancers [19,24]. This extrapulmonary involvement was not found among individuals who developed the traditional late-age-of-onset COPD.

Early serum electrophoresis patterns of AAT indicated three distinct levels of enzyme production, which corresponded to clinical features and suggested an autosomal recessive pattern of inheritance. High producers (normal levels) did not have any particular predisposition to the development of COPD. These individuals were believed to be homozygous for normal alleles of the as yet unidentified gene for AAT. Moderate producers were found to have 40% to 50% of normal serum AAT levels and were considered to be heterozygous with one normal allele and one abnormal allele for the AAT gene. Low producers were found to have absent to approximately 15% of normal levels of serum AAT and were considered to be homozygous for abnormal alleles of the AAT gene. Patients in this low production level category who smoked were the ones who expressed COPD at an early age, although the symptom severity even within this group was wide and provided support for more than one gene mutation leading to disease development [22].

In the 1980s the gene for AAT was identified and localized to chromosome 14 [25,26]. Although more men who were low producers of AAT than women who were low producers of AAT were affected by early-onset COPD, this difference was attributed to gender differences in smoking patterns for the past 60 years rather than to the possibility of an X-linked recessive form of the genetic disorder [19]. Further exploration of the deficiency resulted in the discovery that although mutations of the AAT gene could be found in all races and ethnicities, the enzyme deficiency was most common among whites of Northern European ancestry [27–30]. The manifestations of the deficiency were also noted to be more severe among this group.

In the 1990s great strides were made in identifying different mutations or polymorphisms of the AAT gene, leading to different severities of the disease. Currently, 75 different variations in the AAT gene alleles have been described [19,31], of which 5 combinations seem to have the most significant known clinical relevance (Table 1). Some seem more or less benign, whereas others are associated with varying degrees of enzyme deficiency, early-onset disease in the presence of a smoking history, and shortened lifespan.

Approximately 100,000 Americans have severe AAT deficiency and many more have mild to moderate deficiencies [32]. One in 100 European Americans carries one mutated allele and the incidence of enzyme deficiency leading to disease expression is approximately 1 in 5000 [2]. Of the clinically relevant allele mutations, individuals who are homozygous for the Z/Z mutation have the most severe COPD disease expression [33,34]. New work looking at individuals who have two different mutations of the AAT gene alleles (compound heterozygosity) is uncovering even more variation in the expression of genetic COPD [35,36].

Clinical implications

Most carriers of AAT mutations capable of causing enzyme deficiency are unaware of their status, as are many of the individuals who are homozygous for the less severe forms of the deficiency. Although carriers who have moderate serum levels of AAT who smoke are not at risk for early-age-onset COPD, they may well be the majority of the 15% of cigarette smokers who develop COPD at later ages. If this is the case, obtaining an accurate family history for COPD and other respiratory disorders is important for individualizing or targeting respiratory disease prevention and smoking cessation strategies.

The influence of genetic heterozygosity for the various AAT mutations on the development of other respiratory problems is not currently known, although typical asthma with reversible airway obstruction does not seem to be related to this condition [19]. Many clinical questions remain unanswered. A broad-based question to consider is whether the genetic condition of any level of AAT deficiency contributes to or increases the risk for development of acute respiratory consequences when other medical conditions or traumas are superimposed.

Lung cancer

Disease overview

Lung cancer is the persistent malignant abnormal cell growth anywhere in the airways or parenchymal tissue of the lungs. Primary lung cancer begins in the lungs; secondary lung cancers are actually malignant diseases of other organs that spread or metastasize into the lungs. Although not the most common malignancy in either men or women, it is the leading cause of cancer deaths in North America for both genders [37].

The increasing incidence of lung cancer in the second half of the twentieth century parallels the cigarette smoking prevalence, identified as the single most common "cause" of lung cancer. Similar to COPD, however, other facts indicate that lung cancer is a disorder in which genetic susceptibility versus genetic resistance interplays with environmental susceptibility and resistance. First, not all smokers develop lung cancer even after many decades of cigarette smoking. Second, both nonsmokers and those who have a minimal smoking history also develop the disease.

Pathophysiology

More than 90% of all primary lung cancers arise from the bronchial epithelium [17]. These cancers are differentiated by cell type as epidermoid (squamous cell), adenocarcinoma, and large cell carcinomas, and are collectively classified as

Table 1
Characteristics associated with the most common α_1-antitrypsin gene mutations

Mutation genotype	Level of serum α_1 antitrypsin (% of normal)	Disease severity
M/S	80	No detectable disease
S/S	50–60	Minimal to no disease expression
M/Z	50–55	Minimal to no disease expression
S/Z	30–35	Pulmonary disease, early age
Z/Z	10–15	Severe COPD, extrapulmonary involvement

non–small cell lung cancers (NSCLC). This class is relatively slow growing and may be present for years before manifestations are observed. Small cell lung cancer (SCLC) is an aggressive epithelial cell type cancer with a rapid generation time and often is metastasized widely at diagnosis.

Like other types of cancer, lung cancer represents a loss of control over cell division at the gene level. Chronic exposure to carcinogens damages the DNA of lung epithelial cells. When this damage remains unrepaired or under-repaired, the result is either the loss of gene functions that serve as ''checkpoints'' and ''guardians'' of well-controlled cell division, or the overexpression of genes that promote cell division even when it is not needed for replacement of dead or damaged normal cells. Carcinogens known to cause this damage and lead to poorly regulated cell growth include many chemicals present in cigarette smoke and other forms of tobacco. Additional known environmental carcinogenic substances associated with lung cancer development include asbestos, beryllium, chromium, coal distillates, cobalt, iron oxide, mustard gas, petroleum distillates, radiation, tar, nickel, uranium, and the industrial pollutants of benzopyrenes and hydrocarbons.

Lung cancers metastasize by direct extension, through the blood, and by lymphatic invasion. Tumors in the bronchial tubes can grow and internally obstruct the airways. Tumors in other areas of lung tissue can enlarge and obstruct airways externally. Tumors in the edges of the lungs spread and can compress lung structures other than the airway, including the alveoli, nerves, blood vessels, and lymph vessels.

The patterns of metastasis depend on the type of tumor cell and the anatomic location of the tumor. Local and distant lymph nodes are invaded. Blood-borne metastasis is attributable to tumor invasion of the pulmonary blood vessels, allowing tumor emboli to spread to distant body areas (typically bone, liver, brain, and adrenal glands).

Clinical picture

Typically, the person who has lung cancer presents as a 50- to 60-year-old who has hoarseness, cough, sputum production, hemoptysis, shortness of breath, or change in endurance. Often a significant unplanned weight loss has occurred as the work of ventilation uses more energy than is derived from caloric intake. Chest pain that is localized or unilateral may be present as may sensations of fullness, tightness, or

pressure in the chest. Piercing chest pain or pleuritic pain may occur on inspiration; subscapular pain radiating to the arm results from tumor invasion of nerve plexuses in advanced disease.

Persistent chills, fever, and cough may be related to pneumonitis or bronchitis and are associated with obstruction of the bronchi. Hemoptysis is a late finding. The position of the trachea may be displaced from midline if a mass is present in the area. Additional manifestations, known as paraneoplastic syndromes, may be present with SCLC and are caused by various hormones, antigens, or enzymes secreted by tumor cells. These include edema formation, gynecomastia, hypercalcemia, hypoglycemia, syndrome of inappropriate antidiuretic hormone (SIADH), and a Cushingoid appearance.

Without treatment lung cancer is lethal, with the most common causes of death being respiratory failure and pneumonia. Because of frequent presence of advanced disease at the time of diagnosis, the overall long-term survival rate for lung cancer remains low.

Genetic features

At first glance, lung cancer would seem to belong only on the environmental side of the gene–environment interaction continuum (see Fig. 1). This observation is supported by the dose–response relationship seen between cigarette smoking and disease development, with heavier smokers having a greater incidence of lung cancer. Differences in lung cancer incidence by race, gender, familial association, and smoking history do exist, however, and have driven the exploration for identifying possible genetic factors involved in the gene–environment interactions for lung cancer development.

The puzzlement of why some heavy smokers never develop lung cancer while some lighter smokers and nonsmokers do begs a genetic explanation. Early studies examining this phenomenon posed an increased genetic susceptibility based on alterations in how an individual handled the environmental exposure to carcinogens, including those in cigarette smoke [38–41]. This line of reasoning focused on the body's enzyme systems that metabolize and detoxify noxious agents taken into the body, thus reducing overall tissue exposure to such substances, including potentially carcinogenic agents. Having highly active detoxifying systems thus would be a genetic resistance factor. Major known families of metabolizing and detoxifying enzymes include the cytochrome P450

(CYP) system, glutathione S-transferase system, and the myeloperoxidase system, among others.

The CYP system has been most extensively investigated and has been found to have many gene variations (polymorphisms) among individuals that change its activity and efficiency. For individuals who have variations in the gene that make this enzyme system less effective at metabolism and detoxification, there is less genetic resistance to the increased environmental susceptibility of exposure to the carcinogens in cigarette smoke. For those individuals whose gene variations of the CPY enzyme system nearly eliminate this system's capacity to detoxify any carcinogen, even minimal exposure to inhalation irritants might lead to lung cancer development.

Another individual difference that leads to varying risk for lung cancer among smokers is the ability to repair the cell damage acquired by exposure to carcinogens. DNA repair enzymes exist to repair base substitutions occurring as a result of errors during DNA replication. These repair systems also repair DNA damage and mutations occurring from exposure to carcinogens. The level of accuracy and activity of DNA repair systems is genetically determined and known mutations in these systems increase personal risk for general and specific cancer development [41,42].

Differences in racial and gender incidences in lung cancer among both smokers and nonsmokers also support a genetic factor favoring lung cancer development. Lung cancer has a higher incidence and greater mortality in nonwhites. The incidence is highest among African Americans and Native Hawaiians at lower levels of smoking and lowest among Japanese Americans and Latinos [43].

Demographic data have indicated female smokers to be at higher risk for lung cancer than male smokers. Explanations for this difference have included that women have smaller lung volumes and, therefore, the amount of carcinogens per cigarette smoked is spread over a smaller area, concentrating the dose. Other studies report that gender differences and variation in the activity of the glutathione S-transferase enzyme system correlate strongly to lung cancer development among women who smoke [44]. In addition, variance in lung cancer development among non-smoking women exists and suggests still different genetic susceptibilities. In examining the family histories of nonsmoking women and development of lung cancer, nonsmoking women who have a mother or sibling who have lung cancer are more than twice as likely to develop lung cancer themselves compared with nonsmoking women who have no first-degree relatives who have lung cancer [45]. These findings show no correlation to female size differences and differences in levels of estrogen as possible influences on lung cancer development.

More recent evidence supports the possibility that genetic differences in cell division regulation (cell cycle regulation) may be the genetic susceptibility link for lung cancer development. A major gene involved in cell cycle regulation is the Tp53 suppressor gene. Mutations in the alleles of this gene are known to increase the susceptibility to a wide variety of cancers both with and without exposure to environmental risks. Examination of the expression of this gene and its product indicates a strong predisposition to lung cancer development among smokers and nonsmokers [46,47].

The observation that lung cancers generally arise from epithelial tissues stimulated research into exploring differences in those pathways using growth factors that promote the growth of epithelial cells as altering the risk for lung cancer. The specific growth factor known to affect the growth of lung cancer cells is epidermal growth factor (EGF) and its receptor (EGFR). These substances seem to influence the development of some types of lung cancers even among non-smokers [48].

Clinical implications

Although cigarette smoking continues to be the primary cause of lung cancer, genetic differences affect individual susceptibility to the disease to some extent, even among nonsmokers. The gene–environment interaction promoting lung cancer development is complex, with the environmental susceptibility of cigarette smoking ever present. Major strategies in the reduction of risk for lung cancer are to teach about smoking avoidance and smoking cessation.

The correlation between cigarette smoking and lung cancer development is so strong that any thought of lung cancer susceptibility among non-smokers may be forgotten by health care professionals. As a result, the diagnosis of lung cancer among nonsmokers often occurs late in the disease. Given the information discovered in the last 2 decades that gene variation promoting lung cancer development exists, the possibility of lung cancer for any patient, regardless of smoking status, should be considered whenever clinical responses to treatment of respiratory problems fail to meet expectations. For example, the patient who has repeated episodes of pneumonia or the one in whom all manifestations of pneumonia fail to resolve with conventional treatment may actually have either lung cancer alone or pneumonia and lung cancer. For any patient who has a respiratory problem, obtaining family information for all types of pulmonary disease should be a part of initial history.

Acute respiratory distress syndrome

Disease overview

Acute respiratory distress syndrome (ARDS) is acute lung injury that is associated with severe trauma, systemic infection, or sustained hypoperfusion. Acute lung injury progressing to ARDS can be the result of direct lung injuries, such as pneumothorax or artificial/mechanical hyperventilation. ARDS occurs even in the absence of underlying or pre-event pulmonary pathology. Although the mechanism and causes of ARDS vary, the common pathology is damage to the capillary endothelial cells and alveolar epithelial cells. ARDS is manifested as respiratory failure and has a mortality rate of 50% to 60% even when intensive interventions are used. Other terms for ARDS include noncardiogenic pulmonary edema, adult respiratory distress syndrome, and shock lung. Although once believed to be purely a result of environmental factors, the role of the individual's inflammatory responses also influence the degree to which the problem develops and the extent of recovery.

Pathophysiology

In addition to trauma, sepsis, and shock, known causes of ARDS include brain injury, fat and amniotic fluid emboli, inhalation of toxic gases, excessive oxygen therapy, aspiration of highly acidic or highly basic substances, multiple transfusions, prolonged cardiopulmonary bypass, near drowning in fresh water, and severe acute pancreatitis. Some causes involve direct injury to lung tissue; others do not directly involve the respiratory system. For example, any condition that leads to cerebral hypoxia or a sudden increase in intracranial pressure can cause massive sympathetic discharge, leading to systemic vasoconstriction with movement of large volumes of blood into pulmonary circulation. Intrapulmonary hydrostatic pressure increase leads to fluid shifts and lung injury. Despite different causes of lung injury in ARDS, a systemic inflammatory response is the common pathway in its development. Manifestations of ARDS are thus similar regardless of the cause.

The major site of injury in the lung is the alveolar–capillary membrane, which is normally permeable to only small molecules. The interstitium of the lung normally remains relatively dry, but in patients who have ARDS, lung fluid increases and contains a high level of proteins. At the tissue level, the problem basic to ARDS is the large inflammatory responses set into motion by direct or indirect lung injury that can occur with or without the presence of infectious microorganisms. With direct lung injury, both type I pneumocytes and type II pneumocytes can be severely damaged or destroyed, along with capillary damage. This damage, along with the tissue macrophages and circulating leukocytes, triggers capillary leak syndrome, which allows protein and cells to escape from the blood vessels into lung tissues. Some of the leaked plasma proteins include thromboplastin, increasing clot production, and decreasing fibrinolysis. As a result, myriad small emboli are formed and remain in the lung. Disseminated intravascular coagulation plays a role in some patients.

Other changes occur in the alveoli and respiratory bronchioles. The type II pneumocyte is responsible for producing surfactant, a substance that maintains lung tissue compliance, reduces excessive recoil, and prevents alveolar collapse. Surfactant activity is reduced in ARDS either because type II pneumocytes are damaged or because the surfactant is diluted by excess lung fluids. As a result, the alveoli become unstable and tend to collapse. Collapsed alveoli can no longer participate in gas exchange and edema forms around terminal airways, which are compressed, closed, and susceptible to destruction or necrosis. Lung volume is further reduced, and there is even less compliance. As fluid continues to leak in more lung areas, fluid, protein, and blood cells collect in the alveoli and the interstitial space between the alveoli. Lymph channels are compressed and ineffective. Poorly ventilated alveoli receive blood but cannot oxygenate it, increasing the physiologic shunt. Hypoxemia and ventilation–perfusion mismatch result.

Clinical picture

The typical patient who has ARDS at first presents with only mild to moderate respiratory symptoms that gradually worsen, resulting in increased work of breathing. As breathing becomes more difficult, hyperpnea, grunting respiration, cyanosis, pallor, and intercostal or substernal retractions occur. Diaphoresis, change in mental status, tachycardia, and dysrhythmias are common as hypoxia worsens. No abnormal lung sounds are present on auscultation because the edema of ARDS occurs first in the interstitial spaces and not in the airways.

The diagnosis of ARDS is established by a lowered Pao_2 value, determined by ABG measurements. Because a widening alveolar oxygen gradient (increased fraction of inspired oxygen [Fio_2] does not lead to increased Pao_2 levels) develops with increased shunting of blood, the need for higher levels of oxygen occurs although the patient may not respond to high concentrations of oxygen and often needs intubation and mechanical ventilation. The chest radiograph usually shows diffuse haziness or a whited-out (ground-glass) appearance of the lung. The pulmonary capillary wedge pressure is usually low to normal.

Pulmonary fibrosis with progression occurs after 10 days in some patients. This phase is irreversible and is often called late or chronic ARDS. Individuals who develop this stage and survive it have some permanent lung damage and may be ventilator dependent for weeks to months. Some patients may not wean and remain dependent on mechanical ventilation for the rest of their lives.

Genetic features

Although sepsis and other pulmonary infections seem to increase the risk for development of ARDS when other conditions are present, the role of the inflammatory responses is directly related to the ultimate outcome of this problem [38,49,50]. The longer the inflammatory responses continue and the more fluid that accumulates within lungs, the more likely some degree of pulmonary fibrosis will occur.

Individual variation in the normally protective inflammatory responses has been observed in all aspects of the process of inflammation. The sequence starts with identification of the presence of tissue injury or microbial invasion, progresses to initial stimulation of proinflammatory cytokines and cells, then to direct and indirect actions of these products in changing the expression of various enhancing and suppressing pathways, to the final phases of cellular healing and normalization of function [50]. The genes regulating inflammatory responses are many and work in

a complicated interactive set of pathways to ensure adequate protection from the process while, at the same time, avoiding the consequences of inflammatory excesses. Such gene products include the various cytokines, cytokine receptors, activating and inhibitory enzymes, growth factors, and signaling substances to activate energy-producing pathways [51]. Just like the cytochrome P450 enzyme system, the genetic pathways involved in evoking and regulating inflammatory responses are subject to mutations that unbalance the regulation, allowing some individuals to be hyperresponders to inflammatory triggers. Such individuals are theoretically at increased genetic susceptibility for extended and tissue-damaging inflammatory responses, which are known to stimulate excessive fibrosis and scar tissue formation.

Processing of collagen during inflammation seems to play a role in whether or not the process leads to irreversible fibrosis. The continuing presence of some forms of collagen or collagen metabolites allows a more constant signaling of proinflammatory factors. One study was able to find an association between increased blood levels of specific biomarkers for collagen metabolism and more rapid progression through the stages of ARDS and development of fibrosis [52]. Collagen and its metabolites represent gene products. Although the source or trigger for excessive collagen metabolism may not rest within the collagen genes, it is likely that a genetic variation in some product involved in inflammation leads to excessive transcription of collagen genes.

Clinical implications

Health care professionals involved in critical care are familiar with the conditions that lead to ARDS development and are vigilant in the early identification of its manifestations. That some individuals rapidly progress to the fibrotic stage and others recover before fibrosis occurs is a clinical riddle often attributed to differences in either the severity of the initiating event or the quality of care provided. Although these factors do influence the ultimate outcome of ARDS in a major way, so does the individual patient's genetic makeup with regard to inflammation.

At the present time, it is possible to identify some differences just by history. For example, those individuals who develop high fevers in response to relatively low-level infections are considered to be super responders. This distinction, however, does not mean that such individuals also produce prolonged or excessive responses leading to fibrosis and tissue damage. Currently there is no clinical test that identifies individuals who have increased susceptibility to ARDS development and permanent fibrosis before the syndrome begins. Once again, the future of individualized health problem management may be possible when the meanings of the pathways of inflammatory regulation are fully characterized and the multitude of polymorphisms in the genes responsible for inflammation is known. Microarray gene analysis is most likely to provide a means of identifying genetically susceptible individuals before ARDS actually develops.

Infectious disorders

Tuberculosis

Disease overview

Infection as a general process has been known for more than a century; however, specific cellular events and mechanisms of infection are just now coming to light. Investigation of infection mechanisms has led to the discovery that many diverse human illnesses, such as coronary artery disease, rheumatoid arthritis, type I diabetes mellitus, and peptic ulcer disease, actually are sequelae of infection. As discussed earlier, susceptibility to infection in the presence of any given microorganism is not equal among humans. Host inflammatory responses and immune responses, both of which are regulated by gene activity, are responsible for prevention of and recovery from infection. Both infection and prevention of infection require distinct interactions between the invading bacteria and the host at the cellular and subcellular levels.

Bacterial infection is the most common cause of disease, sepsis, and death worldwide, although infection with other types of microorganisms also is a serious health problem [53]. Tuberculosis (TB), caused by *Mycobacterium tuberculosis*, is the most common infectious disease today, infecting approximately one third of the world's population [54]. Exposure to the microorganism is a prerequisite for infection; however, there is huge variance in expression of the disease among exposed and infected individuals.

Pathophysiology

TB is a highly communicable disease caused by *M tuberculosis*. This organism is a nonmoving, slow-growing, acid-fast rod transmitted by way of aerosolization.

Airborne droplets are inhaled by others and may multiply when the bacillus reaches the bronchi or alveoli. An exudative response occurs, causing a nonspecific pneumonitis. With the development of acquired immunity, further multiplication of bacilli is controlled and the lesions typically resolve with little or no residual. A small percentage of individuals who are initially infected, however, will acquire the disease (5% to 15%) [17].

Cell-mediated immunity develops 2 to 10 weeks after infection and is manifested by a significant reaction to a tuberculin test. This primary infection may never appear on a radiograph.

The granulomatous inflammation created by the bacillus in the lung is surrounded by collagen, fibroblasts, and lymphocytes. Caseation necrosis (necrotic tissue being turned into a granular mass) occurs in the center of the lesion. This area, a Ghon tubercle, may be evident on chest radiograph as the primary lesion. Areas of caseation then undergo degeneration and fibrosis. Necrotic areas may form calcifications or may liquefy and empty into a bronchus. The evacuated area then becomes a cavity but bacilli continue to grow in this area and spread by way of lymph nodes into new areas of the lung.

Lesions may progress by direct extension with rapid bacilli proliferation and marked exudate formation. Lesions may extend through the pleura, resulting in pleural and pericardial effusions.

Hematogenous or miliary TB occurs when a large number of organisms enter the bloodstream and the disease is spread throughout the body. The brain, meninges, liver, and kidney or bone marrow are commonly involved as a result of spread through the blood.

There is usually an asymptomatic interval after the primary infection that lasts for years or decades before clinical symptoms develop. Although infected, an individual is not infectious to others until symptoms of disease occur. Secondary TB occurs in a previously infected person and is a reactivation of the primary disease.

Clinical picture

TB has an insidious onset, and many individuals are not aware of symptoms until the disease is well advanced. Common general manifestations include a persistent cough, weight loss, anorexia, night sweats, hemoptysis, shortness of breath, fever, and chills. These nonspecific manifestations may have been present for weeks or months. The sputum is mucopurulent sputum and may be streaked with blood. Chest tightness and a dull, aching chest pain may accompany the cough. Some people recover from active disease with only prolonged rest and nutrition, whereas others die of the disease even with appropriate treatment. In addition, drug-resistant strains of the microorganism are becoming more common.

A diagnosis of TB is suggested by the manifestations, a positive purified protein derivative test, and a positive smear for acid-fast bacillus. Diagnosis is confirmed by polymerase chain reaction assays to rapidly identify specific mycobacteria. Other genetic tests may be performed to identify drug-resistant strains of the organism.

Genetic features

Exposure of humans to the TB organism occurs frequently and exposure to other bacteria is constant in the natural environment. When disease results from bacterial invasion, the action represents either unsuccessful host protection or successful evasion of host protection by the bacteria. General observations of TB disease development after substantial exposure or infection with the organism reveal groups of individuals who are more resistant to disease development, groups of individuals who are less resistant to disease development, and groups of individuals who demonstrate expected levels of disease resistance. This variance can be explained by differences in the microorganism, differences in host defenses, and the combination of host and organism differences.

To prevent disease after exposure/infection with an organism, the human host must be able to distinguish invading bacteria from self-cells and cell products and also must be able to mount appropriate defensive actions against bacteria without harming normal body cells and tissues. Cells of the human host must be able to communicate that invasion has occurred and must be able to coordinate responses tailored to the level of threat posed by the specific invader. For the invasion to develop into infection, the invading bacteria must successfully evade multiple host defenses.

Interaction between invading bacteria and human body cells is required for successful infection on the part of the bacteria and successful prevention of infection on the part of host cells. Key areas of interaction are the membranes and membrane molecules of the host cells and those of the invading bacteria.

The fruit fly has four cell surface receptors, termed Toll receptors, that have continuing roles in protecting the fruit fly from bacterial infection. Identical genes and receptors have been discovered in human cells and seem to have similar functions to prevent or control infection. More than 10 human receptors, termed Toll-like receptors (TLRs), have been identified and characterized. These TLRs assist in the key activity of pathogen recognition to induce inflammatory and immune protective actions to prevent infectious disease expression. Individuals who have altered TLR numbers or reduced TLR activity as a result of genetic polymorphisms have reduced protection against TB and other infectious diseases [55]. Such a condition represents a loss of host genetic resistance. In addition some bacteria are able to avoid host protective responses by inactivating host TLRs and inducing programmed cell death (apoptosis) in macrophages and other inflammatory cells [56]. This condition represents an increase in environmental susceptibility.

When TB enters host lung cells, a degree of sanctuary has been achieved. The invaders are now safe from the reach of antibodies and phagocytes. Usually when a bacterium is brought into a macrophage, a phagosome is formed. The phagosome then fuses with a lysosome to form a phagolysosome. This step is key to bacterial destruction because the degrading enzymes are confined to the lysosome. Phagocytized TB organisms escape this destruction by preventing phagosomal fusion with the lysosome. Then the organism can use the host cell cytoplasm as a breeding ground. The *M tuberculosis* thus enters macrophages and actually uses this site as a sanctuary for many years by changing the metabolism of the infected macrophage. This change prevents a normal phagosome coating called TACO (tryptophan-aspartate containing coat protein) from detaching. When TACO remains attached, phagolysosomes do not form. In addition, retention of TACO hides the *Mycobacterium*-infected macrophage from destruction by cell-mediated immune responses [57].

Although these changes in the host genetic susceptibility and resistance to TB disease development and the acquired genetic differences in the organism that enable it to bypass host defenses can be traced to one type of response, other genetic polymorphisms also contribute to reduced resistance to the disease. For example, examination of families who have increased genetic susceptibility to TB revealed variation in alleles of a gene called NRAMP1, natural resistance–associated macrophage protein [58]. Variation in the same gene was found to be a risk factor for the development of pediatric TB disease [59]. In addition, racial differences in susceptibility to TB disease have also been noted. The issues of genetic and environmental resistance to TB disease and genetic and environmental susceptibility to TB disease are thus complex and involve gene differences in the host and the microorganism [60].

Clinical implications

TB can be considered a model for many infectious diseases of bacterial origin because of the known variation in genetic resistance and susceptibility associated with it. Indeed several of the pathways to reduced resistance are also found to reduce resistance to other bacteria [56].

At this point, little is known about general host genetic resistance and susceptibility to common bacterial infections, even among health care workers. Given the state of genetic changes in bacteria, however, resulting in greater virulence and more drug resistance, all people are more susceptible to bacterial infections than in previous decades. With the advent of effective antibiotic therapy and resultant reduction in deaths from uncontrolled infection and sepsis, some medical asepsis practices have not been as strictly used or enforced as they were before antibiotic therapy. Now that more bacteria are developing drug resistance, strategies in addition to antibiotic therapy are needed to control infection spread. Medical asepsis practices, especially handwashing, must be dragged out, dusted off, and consistently applied in all health care settings and in other environments where infectious organisms can gain a foothold, such as homes, schools, places of employment, and residential facilities.

Summary

The expression of many common respiratory disorders represents a gene–environment interaction in which susceptibility is unbalanced by resistance. For those disorders with a strong genetic susceptibility component, such as cystic fibrosis and COPD as a result of a deficiency of α_1-antitrypsin, environmental resistance strategies can help to restore some balance to modify disease expression. Such strategies can include smoking cessation, avoidance of inhalation irritants, avoidance of airborne or droplet infectious agents, adherence to prescribed drug therapies, and engaging in health-promoting activities. For those disorders that have a strong environmental susceptibility component, the focus of health care and prevention must still be on implementation of environmental resistance strategies because genetic resistance cannot be changed. Health care professionals need to remain cognizant of the possibility for increased genetic susceptibility to respiratory diseases even when the individual has no known environmental risk factors. This awareness may allow earlier intervention for some health problems, when better responses to interventions are more likely.

References

[1] Workman ML. The cellular basis of bacterial infection. Crit Care Nurs Clin North Am 2003;15(1): 1–11.
[2] Nussbaum R, McInnes R, Willard H. Thompson & Thompson: genetics in medicine. 7th edition. Philadelphia: W.B. Saunders; 2007.
[3] Pier GB, Grout M, Zaidi T, et al. Salmonella typhi uses CFTR to enter intestinal epithelial cells. Nature 1998;393:79–82.
[4] Quinton PM. Physiological basis of cystic fibrosis: a historical perspective. Physiol Rev 1999; 79(Suppl):S3–22.
[5] Andersen DH. Cystic fibrosis of the pancreas and its relation to celiac disease. Am J Dis Child 1938;56: 344–99.
[6] Andersen DH, Hodges R. Celiac syndrome. V. Genetics of cystic fibrosis of the pancreas with a consideration of the etiology. Am J Dis Child 1946;72: 62–80.
[7] di Sant'agnese PA, Darling RC, Perera GA, et al. Abnormal electrolyte composition of sweat in cystic fibrosis of the pancreas. Pediatrics 1953;12:549–63.
[8] Thomaidis TS, Arey JB. The intestinal lesions in cystic fibrosis of the pancreas. J Pediatr 1963;63:444–53.
[9] Holsclaw DS, Perelmutter AD, Jockin H, et al. Genital abnormalities in males with cystic fibrosis: an emerging problem. J Urol 1971;106:568–74.
[10] Tsui L-C, Buchwald M, Barker D, et al. Cystic fibrosis locus defined by a genetically linked polymorphic DNA marker. Science 1985;230:1054–7.
[11] Kerem B, Rommens JM, Buchanan JA, et al. Identification of the cystic fibrosis gene: genetic analysis. Science 1989;245:1073–80.
[12] Reddy MM, Quinton PM. Control of dynamic CFTR selectivity by glutamate and ATP in epithelial cells. Nature 2003;423:756–60.
[13] Kulczycki L, Kostuch M, Bellanti J. A clinical perspective of cystic fibrosis and new genetic findings: relationship of CFTR mutations to

genotype-phenotype manifestations. Am J Med Genet 2003;116:262–7.

[14] Kerem E, Corey M, Kerem B, et al. The relation between genotype and phenotype in cystic fibrosis—analysis of the most common mutation (delta-F508). N Engl J Med 1990;323:1517–22.

[15] Grossman S, Grossman LC. Pathophysiology of cystic fibrosis: implications for critical care nurses. Crit Care Nurse 2005;25(4):46–51.

[16] Gardner J. What you need to know about cystic fibrosis. Nursing 2007;37(7):52–5.

[17] Kumar V, Abbas A, Fausto N. Robbins and Cotran pathologic basis of disease. 7th edition. Philadelphia: W.B. Saunders; 2005.

[18] Chappell S, Daly L, Morgan K, et al. Cryptic haplotypes of SERPINA1 confer susceptibility to chronic obstructive pulmonary disease. Hum Mutat 2006;27: 103–9.

[19] Coakley R, Taggart C, O'Neill S, et al. alpha(sub1)-antitrypsin deficiency: biological answers to clinical questions. Am J Med Sci 2001;321(1):33–41.

[20] Kueppers F, Briscoe WA, Bearn AG. Hereditary deficiency of serum alpha-1-antitrypsin. Science 1964; 146:1678–9.

[21] Laurell CB, Eriksson S. The serum of alpha-1-antitrypsin in families with hypo-alpha-1-antitrypsinemia. Clin Chim Acta 1965;11:395–8.

[22] Tarkoff MP, Kueppers F, Miller WF. Pulmonary emphysema and alpha-1-antitrypsin deficiency. Am J Med 1968;45:220–8.

[23] Guenter CA, Welch MH, Hammarsten JF. Alpha-1-antitrypsin deficiency and pulmonary emphysema. Annu Rev Med 1971;22:283–92.

[24] Crystal RG. Alpha-1-antitrypsin deficiency, emphysema, and liver disease: genetic basis and strategies for therapy. J Clin Invest 1990;85:1343–52.

[25] Darlington GJ, Astrin KH, Muirhead SP, et al. Assignment of human alpha-1-antitrypsin to chromosome 14 by somatic cell hybrid analysis. Proc Natl Acad Sci U S A 1982;79:870–3.

[26] Cox DW, Billingsley GD, Mansfield T, et al. DNA restriction-site polymorphisms associated with the alpha-1-antitrypsin gene. Am J Hum Genet 1987; 41:891–906.

[27] Curiel DT, Vogelmeier C, Hubbard RC, et al. Molecular basis of alpha-1-antitrypsin deficiency and emphysema associated with the alpha-1-antitrypsin M(Mineral Springs) allele. Mol Cell Biol 1990;10: 47–56.

[28] DeCroo S, Kamboh MI, Ferrell RE. Population genetics of alpha-1-antitrypsin polymorphism in US whites, US blacks and African blacks. Hum Hered 1991;41:215–21.

[29] Blanco I, Bustillo EF, Rodriguez MC. Distribution of alpha-1-antitrypsin PI S and PI Z frequencies in countries outside Europe: a meta-analysis. Clin Genet 2001;60:431–41.

[30] de Serres FJ, Blanco I, Fernandez-Bustillo E. Genetic epidemiology of alpha-1-antitrypsin deficiency in North America and Australia/New Zealand: Australia, Canada, New Zealand and the United States of America. Clin Genet 2003;64:382–97.

[31] Faber JP, Poller W, Weidinger S, et al. Identification and DNA sequence analysis of 15 new alpha-1-antitrypsin variants, including two Pi* Q alleles and one deficient Pi* M allele. Am J Hum Genet 1994;55: 1113–21.

[32] Stoller JK. Clinical features and natural history of severe alpha(sub1)-antitrypsin deficiency. Chest 1997;111(6):123s–8s.

[33] Harrison HH, Miller KL, Whitington PF. Improved detection, via ISO-DALT two-dimensional electrophoresis, of 'low Z expressor' individuals with alpha-1-antitrypsin MZ phenotype. Clin Chem 1990; 36:1850–1.

[34] Seri M, Magi B, Cellesi C, et al. Molecular characterization of the P and I variants of alpha-1-antitrypsin. Int J Clin Lab Res 1992;22:119–21.

[35] Klaassen CH, deMetz M, van Aarssen Y, et al. Alpha(1)-antitrypsin deficiency as a result of compound heterozygosity for the Z and M(Heerlen) alleles. Clin Chem 2001;47(5):978–9.

[36] Dahl M, Tybjaerg-Hansen A, Lange P, et al. Change in lung function and morbidity from chronic obstructive pulmonary disease in alpha-1-antitrypsin MZ heterozygotes: a longitudinal study of the general population. Ann Intern Med 2002;136:270–9.

[37] American Cancer Society. Cancer facts and figures 2007. Report No. 01-300M-No. 5008.07. Atlanta: American Cancer Society; 2007.

[38] Warburton D, Oliver R. Coordination of genetic, epigenetic, and environmental factors in lung development, injury, and repair. Chest 1997;111(6):119S–22S.

[39] Spitz MR, Wei Q, Li G, et al. Genetic susceptibility to tobacco carcinogenesis. Cancer Invest 1999;17(8): 645–59.

[40] Laforest L, Wikman H, Benhamou S, et al. CYP2D6 gene polymorphism in Caucasian smokers: lung cancer susceptibility and phenotype-genotype relationships. Eur J Cancer 2000;36(14):1825–32.

[41] Kiyohara C, Otsu A, Shirakawa T, et al. Genetic polymorphisms and lung cancer susceptibility: a review. Lung Cancer 2002;37:241–56.

[42] Wu X, Zhao H, Suk R, et al. Genetic susceptibility to tobacco-related cancer. Oncogene 2004;23(38): 6500–23.

[43] Haiman CA, Stram DO, Wilkens LR, et al. Ethnic and racial differences in the smoking-related risk of lung cancer. N Engl J Med 2006;354:333–42.

[44] Tang DL, Rundle A, Warburton D, et al. Association between both genetic and environmental biomarkers and lung cancer: evidence of a greater risk of lung cancer in women smokers. Carcinogenesis 1998;19(11):1949–53.

[45] Wu AH, Fontham ET, Reynolds P. Family history of cancer and risk of lung cancer among lifetime nonsmoking women in the United States. Am J Epidemiol 1996;143:535–42.

[46] Hwang SJ, Cheng LS, Lozano G, et al. Lung cancer risk in germline p53 mutation carriers: association between an inherited cancer predisposition, cigarette smoking, and cancer risk. Hum Genet 2003;113(3): 238–43.

[47] Zhang X, Mioa X, Guo Y, et al. Genetic polymorphisms in cell cycle regulatory genes MDM2 and TP53 are associated with susceptibility to lung cancer. Hum Mutat 2006;27(1):110–7.

[48] Pao W, Miller V, Zakowski M, et al. EGF receptor gene mutations are common in lung cancers from "never smokers" and are associated with sensitivity of tumors to gefitinib and erlotinib. Proc Natl Acad Sci U S A 2004;101:13306–11.

[49] Bauer TT, Ewig S, Rodloff AC, et al. Acute respiratory distress syndrome and pneumonia: A comprehensive review of clinical data. Clin Infect Dis 2006;43(6):748–56.

[50] Winkelman C. Inflammation and genomics in the critical care unit. Crit Care Nurs Clin North Am 2008;20(2):213–21.

[51] Jiang D, Liang J, Fan J, et al. Regulation of lung injury and repair by Toll-like receptors and hyaluronan. Nat Med 2005;11:1173–9.

[52] Farjanel J, Hartmann DJ, Guidet B, et al. Four markers of collagen metabolism as possible indicators of disease in the adult respiratory distress syndrome. Am Rev Respir Dis 1993;147(5):1091–9.

[53] Strauss EJ, Falkow S. Microbial pathogenesis: genomics and beyond. Science 1997;276(5313):707–13.

[54] World Health Organization: Global tuberculosis control. WHO Report 2005. World Health Organization; 2000.

[55] Khor CC, Chapman SJ, Vannberg FO, et al. A Mal functional variant is associated with protection against invasive pneumococcal disease, bacteremia, malaria and tuberculosis. Nat Genet 2007;39:523–8.

[56] Hsu LC, Park JM, Zhong K, et al. The protein kinase PKR is required for macrophage apoptosis after activation of Toll-like receptor 4. Nature 2004;428:341–5.

[57] Pieters J. Entry and survival of pathogenic mycobacteria in macrophages. Microbes Infect 2001;3(3): 249–55.

[58] Greenwood CM, Fujiwara TM, Boothroyd LJ, et al. Linkage of tuberculosis to chromosome 2q35 loci, including NRAMP1, in a large aboriginal Canadian family. Am J Hum Genet 2000;67(2):405–16.

[59] Malik S, Abel L, Tooker H, et al. Alleles of the NRAMP1 gene are risk factors for pediatric tuberculosis disease. Proc Natl Acad Sci U S A 2005; 102(34):12183–8.

[60] Abel L, Casanova J. Genetic predisposition to clinical tuberculosis: bridging the gap between simple and complex inheritance. Am J Hum Genet 2000; 67:274–7.

ELSEVIER
SAUNDERS

Crit Care Nurs Clin N Am 20 (2008) 191–201

CRITICAL CARE
NURSING CLINICS
OF NORTH AMERICA

Hereditary Hemochromatosis: Pathophysiology, Diagnosis, and Management

Christopher Fowler, PhD, RN, ACNP[a,b*]

[a]Transplant Services, Methodist Dallas Medical Center, 1441 North Beckley Avenue,
4th Floor, Service Building, Dallas, TX 75203, USA
[b]School of Nursing, University of Texas at Arlington, 411 South Nedderman Drive, Pickard Hall,
Arlington, TX 76019-0407, USA

Until slightly more than a decade ago, hereditary hemochromatosis (HH) was believed to be a rare condition. With the discovery of several genetic mutations that lead to excessive iron absorption and storage, research has identified a higher prevalence and increased our understanding of the disease. Although multiple genetic mutations can occur that result in iron overload, this article addresses HH in adults resulting solely from mutations on the HFE gene.

HH is the most common identified genetic disorder in the white population [1]. It results from an inborn error of iron metabolism characterized by increased intestinal iron absorption despite adequate and even excessive iron stores, leading to progressive iron accumulation in the body with irreversible damage to various organs [2,3]. Iron levels in HH may reach 10 to 30 times normal [4–6]. It is an autosomal recessive disease and is concentrated in individuals of northern European origin, especially those of Nordic or Celtic ancestry. In this population, the prevalence is close to 1:200 [1]. Although HH is a disease of altered iron metabolism, it is a systemic genetic disease with multisystem involvement because of abnormal iron distribution [5,7].

Excessive body iron can have primary and secondary causes. Primary iron overload results from an inherent defect in iron regulation and continuous overabsorption of iron from the gastrointestinal tract. Iron accumulates in the parenchyma of various organs, particularly in the liver, pancreas, and heart, and eventually causes end-organ damage. HH is the most common cause of primary iron overload [8].

Secondary iron overload results from excessive intake of iron from multiple blood transfusions, parenteral iron administration, dietary intake, or iron supplements. Secondary iron overload can also occur in patients who have chronic disorders of erythropoiesis or hemolytic anemias (such as sideroblastic and sickle-cell anemias and β thalassemia) [5,9].

Hereditary hemochromatosis was first recognized almost 150 years ago by Trousseau as a condition with a triad of symptoms (diabetes, bronze-colored skin, and cirrhosis) associated with hepatic, pancreatic, and integumentary iron overload. The condition was first called hemochromatosis in 1889 by von Recklinghausen and it was first identified as an inherited disorder by Sheldon in 1935. Further explanation of the autosomal recessive genetic transmission was noted in 1976 by Simon and colleagues. In 1996, Feder and colleagues localized the gene responsible for most cases of HH on the short arm of chromosome 6 [5,10,11].

HH was originally known as "idiopathic hemochromatosis" and believed to be a rare idiopathic disorder because the diagnosis relied on the identification of symptoms of end-organ disease. More recently, population-based screening studies have demonstrated a higher prevalence of the disease than was previously recognized [8]. It is now recognized as having a hereditary component

* Methodist Dallas Medical Center, Transplant Services, 1441 North Beckley Avenue, 4th Floor, Service Building, Dallas, TX 75203.
E-mail address: christopher.fowler@sbcglobal.net

attributable to an autosomal recessive inherited disorder of iron absorption and metabolism with excess iron being deposited in the liver, pancreas, heart, joints, and endocrine glands. This iron overload leads to cirrhosis, diabetes, heart failure, arthropathy, and impotence [9,12]. The clinical manifestations of HH are attributable to tissue damage resulting from the accumulation of iron to toxic levels within cells [13]. Because the pathogenesis of HH is now more fully understood and laboratory screening tests are used more frequently, the disease is now more commonly recognized at an earlier stage of its natural history and treatment can begin before end-organ damage has occurred [3].

The HFE gene

The aberrancies found to cause most of the cases of HH are located on the HFE gene, discovered in 1996 and originally named HLA-H [6,14,15]. The gene is localized in hand region 21.3 on the short (p) arm of chromosome 6 [5]. The discovery of the HFE gene and the mutations causing HH provided a tool for screening, estimating prevalence, understanding the natural history and phenotypic expression of HH, and for evaluating liver disease etiology [6].

Two base-pair alterations were originally discovered on the HFE gene and they account for most cases of HH. The first mutation is termed C282Y and comes from a guanine-to-adenine replacement in DNA resulting in the substitution of the amino acid cysteine by tyrosine at position 282. The second mutation is termed H63D and involves the replacement of the amino acid histidine by aspartate at position 63 [5]. Heterozygotes carry the gene but do not have like pairs; homozygotes express like pairs [16].

Homozygosity for the C282Y mutation accounts for most HH cases in white adults and the risk for iron overload is greatest in people who are homozygous for the C282Y mutation. The remaining 10% to 18% of cases seem to be attributable to other genotypes or environmental factors [2,17,18].

Population studies have demonstrated that most patients who have C282Y/H63D compound heterozygosity or H63D homozygosity have normal iron studies. Compound heterozygotes and, less commonly, H63D homozygotes may resemble C282Y homozygotes with mild to moderate iron overload, however [7,13,14]. The frequency of the H63D mutation in the general population ranges from 15% to 20% [18]. The H63D mutation seems

to act synergistically with the C282Y mutation and 2% to 5% of compound heterozygotes have clinical symptoms of HH [1,5,7]. Additionally, the H63D homozygotes often have a potentiator, such as hepatitis C virus or β-thalassemia trait [2].

There are a growing number of less common genetic mutations being identified that may result in iron overload [7]. Other rarer mutations in the HFE gene that have been described include S65C, V53M, V59M, H63H, Q127H, Q283P, P168X, E168Q, E168X, and W169X. These mutations are usually associated with mild iron overload [3,13]. It is likely that other unidentified genes play a role in HH because studies have found populations with HH in which the known HFE mutations do not exist [1].

In the small intestine, the HFE gene is localized within crypt cells. It is theorized that iron status is signaled through HFE and that iron flux across enterocytes is modified based on the HFE mutation. It is also theorized that HFE may exert its effects on iron homeostasis within the liver. Likely, both hepatic and intestinal roles for HFE play a part in phenotypic expression of the disease [6]. Loss of the functional HFE protein as a result of the mutations described above is associated with inappropriately increased iron absorption, resulting in the deposition of iron in parenchymal organs and sequelae of iron overload [2]. Suggested roles for the HFE protein in regulating iron absorption include the ability or inability of HFE to bind with a complex containing transferrin receptor on the enterocytes, facilitation of transferrin-bound iron uptake, or modulation of the expression of hepcidin [5].

It is speculated that individuals possessing mutations of the HFE gene may have been favored by natural selection because they would have enhanced uptake of iron from iron-poor diets, thus minimizing their risk for iron deficiency. This benefit may have been further realized in those who were heterozygotes and were unlikely to develop iron overload, but in whom increased intracellular iron levels might have protected them against infectious agents such as *Yersinia* and *Francisella*, the causative agents of plague and tularemia, respectively [5].

Incidence and prevalence

Hemochromatosis is the most common autosomal recessive disorder among white individuals. The prevalence of HH, however, varies depending on the case definition of the disease [19]. Before the identification of the HFE gene, prevalence of HH was based primarily on phenotypic markers of the diseases (serum ferritin and transferrin saturation) [2]. New definitions are currently being considered. Because of the lack of a consistent definition for HH incidence and prevalence data may differ among studies. The prevalence of cases of HH defined biochemically using iron indices is higher than the prevalence of cases based on identification of HFE genetic mutations [9]. The estimated prevalence of HH is 1 in 200 people to 1 in 250 people in the general population and the worldwide prevalence of HH in people aged 18 to 70 years could range between 1.6 and 5.9 per thousand [19,20].

In northern Europe, about 1 in 8 people carry one copy of the C282Y mutation and are identified as carriers of the disease. The prevalence of homozygous carriers of HFE mutations is 5 to 8 per 1000 among people of European descent [12,14,21]. The prevalence of phenotypically expressed HH is 3 to 4 cases per 1000 people in individuals of northern European descent. In Ireland, C282Y has a homozygosity prevalence of 1 in 83 individuals and more than 20% of the population is heterozygous for that mutation [5,6]. Prevalence is especially high among individuals of Celtic ancestry (the Irish, Scots, and Welsh) [5]. The H63D mutation is common throughout Europe and carried by approximately 25% of the population [12].

The prevalence of C282Y mutation in hemochromatosis decreases from northern to southern Europe with the highest percentage occurring in Britain and the lowest percentage occurring in Italy and Greece. In the general white population, the frequency of carriers of H63D mutation nearly doubles that of carriers of the C282Y mutation (20% versus 10%). Another mutation in the HFE gene (S65C) was described in 1999 by Mura and colleagues, who found that the S65C mutation accounted for nearly 8% of hemochromatosis chromosomes that were neither C282Y nor H63D. Additional studies on the prevalence of the S65C mutation have reported an allele frequency ranging from 1.6% to 5.5% in Caucasians [11].

In the United States white population, approximately 1 in 250 to 300 people is homozygous for the hemochromatosis gene mutation and approximately 8 to 12 people are a carrier for the mutation [4,5,9,15,22]. In the Hemochromatosis and Iron Overload Screening Study (HEIRS), the highest prevalence of homozygosity for C282Y mutation was among non-Hispanic whites (4.4 individuals per 1000). The prevalence of the C282Y/C282Y genotype among other minorities was 1.1 cases per 1000 in Native Americans, 1.2 cases per 10,000 in Pacific Islanders, 1.4 cases per 10,000 in African Americans, 2.7 cases per 10,000 in Hispanics, and 3.9 cases per 10 million in Asians [5,9]. Men are about five times more likely to be diagnosed with HH than women and they develop symptoms from excess iron at a younger age, usually by age 40 [6,23].

The HFE mutation is almost absent in African, Asian, and aboriginal Australasian individuals [24]. Asian adults seem to have lower mean transferrin saturations and higher ferritin levels than white adults. There is evidence that Native Americans are descendants of Asians who migrated to the Americas through a Bering land bridge during the last ice age. The observed and estimated frequencies of C282Y and H63D are significantly lower in Native Americans than in whites [25].

Iron metabolism

Almost all cells require iron for enzymatic function and critical metabolic pathways. As such, iron is central to aerobic metabolism. It is part of the functional groups of most enzymes in the Krebs cycle and is the oxygen-binding component in myoglobin and hemoglobin [5]. Iron also serves as a catalyst for chemical reactions associated with the production of reactive oxygen species, which may lead to oxidative stress and cellular damage; therefore, its concentration must be kept within defined physiologic limits to prevent damage to cell membranes, lipids, proteins, and nucleic acids [5]. Excessive iron promotes atherosclerosis through various mechanisms, including the formation of reactive oxygen species, which in turn increase lipid peroxidation. Lipid peroxidation decreases the bioavailability of nitric oxide causing endothelial dysfunction and accelerated atherosclerosis [26]. There is no effective method for the elimination of excess body iron and iron overload from iatrogenic or idiopathic pathologic causes leads to multiple systemic complications [2,10].

The body of an adult male usually contains 3 to 4 g of iron; women contain slightly less. Two thirds of the body's iron is present in hemoglobin, myoglobin, and iron-containing enzymes, with the remainder in storage forms (ferritin and hemosiderin). The liver is the major site of iron storage [5,27]. Quantitatively, most iron is incorporated into hemoglobin within red blood cells, which are phagocytosed by Kupffer cells and macrophages at the end of their life span with iron being returned to the circulation [10]. The principal way we lose iron is through sloughing of ferritin-containing intestinal cells and menstruation [5]. But it is not through iron loss that we normally regulate iron stores; it is through decreased iron absorption. Under normal circumstances, the small intestine epithelium responds to deficiencies or excesses of iron by increasing or decreasing the amount of iron absorbed using a negative feedback mechanism [6].

Normally, only about 10% of dietary iron is absorbed, approximately 1 mg/d [28]. Intestinal epithelial cells lining the absorptive villi close to the gastroduodenal junction absorb iron. Ferrous iron passes through two cellular membranes to cross the enterocytes into the circulation: (1) the apical membrane and (2) the basolateral membrane. Absorption of iron is facilitated by the low pH, which liberates dietary iron and delivers it in a proton-rich fluid.

Intestinal iron absorption is regulated in response to at least three types of stimuli: (1) mucosal block, (2) stores regulator, and (3) erythropoietic regulator. In the mucosal block phenomenon, enterocytes become refractory to absorbing additional iron after recent dietary intake. The stores regulator mechanism adjusts iron absorption in response to total body iron stores. The erythropoietic regulator adjusts iron absorption in response to the demands of erythropoiesis and functions independent of total body iron stores [22].

Iron is absorbed across the epithelial cells of the proximal small intestine in either a heme or nonheme form. Because iron has the capacity to accept and donate electrons readily, it is converted between ferric (+3) and ferrous (+2) forms easily. Nonheme iron exists primarily in the ferric state and is reduced to the ferrous state by ferric reductase. Ferrous iron uptake from the intestinal lumen into the enterocytes is facilitated by the iron transport protein divalent metal transporter 1 (DMT1). DMT1 also helps erythropoietic cells take in iron [5,10,22].

Once absorbed, iron may be stored as ferritin in the enterocytes or it may cross the enterocyte and be exported into the circulation by another iron transport protein called ferroportin (fpn) [22]. Ferroportin is located along the entire basolateral membrane of enterocytes and is induced by iron deficiency [27]. Ferroportin expression is increased in patients who have HH [2]. Ferroportin is also important in recycling iron by moving it

out of macrophages of the liver, spleen, and bone marrow that have recovered hemoglobin iron by phagocytizing old or damaged red blood cells and returning it to the circulation. The ferroxidase hephaestin, a ceruloplasmin-like protein, promotes the reoxidation of Fe^{++} to Fe^{+++} and facilitates the release of iron from hepatocytes [27]. Transfer across the basolateral membrane seems to be aided by this protein [22].

In the plasma, ferric iron binds to transferrin. Plasma transferrin (Tf) binds iron on the basolateral membrane surface and delivers it to body tissues by way of the glycoprotein transferrin receptor (TfR). Receptor-mediated endocytosis of ferric–transferrin complex follows. It is theorized that the HFE protein interacts with TfR to regulate cellular iron uptake [2,5,10]. Iron is then released by endosomal acidification and transported across the endosomal membrane by DMT1 where it is used for metabolic processes or stored as ferritin [10]. Patients who have HH demonstrate increased DMT1 expression [2].

Ferroportin also binds with hepcidin, a peptide synthesized predominantly in the liver and belonging to the defensins, a family of proteins involved in innate immune defense [29]. Hepcidin is a central regulator of body iron metabolism that acts on small intestinal enterocytes, macrophages, and other body cells to limit iron entry into the plasma [30]. When released into the circulation, hepcidin functions as the hormonal regulator of iron uptake and represses iron absorption. Circulating levels of hepcidin increase when iron bound to transferrin is taken into cells, negatively regulating intestinal iron absorption and the release of iron from enterocytes and macrophages [27]. Normally, hepcidin expression increases with iron overload and decreases with iron depletion, altering the amount of iron absorbed in the intestine. Theoretically, by binding with ferroportin, hepcidin would reduce intestinal iron absorption and decrease the release of cellular iron. Patients who have HH may be hepcidin deficient because of defective intrahepatic signaling mechanisms, however, making them unable to effectively repress iron absorption, even in the face of significant iron overload [6,13,29].

HFE is expressed in body tissues and encodes an MHC class I–like molecule. It binds to β_2-microglobulin and this complex is required for expression on the cell surface. Normally, the HFE/β_2-microglobulin complex binds to transferrin receptor. The C282Y mutation disables the HFE Golgi apparatus and abolishes a disulfide bridge, preventing binding to β₂-microglobulin and subsequent binding with the transferrin receptor. Cell-surface expression is then disrupted, resulting in increased cellular iron uptake by way of receptor-mediated endocytosis [6,12,13,22].

When plasma iron content exceeds the iron-binding capacity of transferrin, parenchymal cells of the liver take up iron. As iron overload progresses, cardiac myocytes, pancreatic acinar cells, and other cells accumulate iron [22]. Once a critical threshold level of hepatic iron is achieved, hepatic stellate cell activation and proliferation occur, resulting in increased collagen synthesis and progression to fibrosis and the development of cirrhosis. The hepatocyte iron concentration that is necessary to induce formation of collagen and progression of fibrosis is dynamic and influenced by other factors. Fibrosis and cirrhosis of the liver are usually associated with a hepatic iron concentration 7 to 10 times normal [10].

Clinical course of the disease

Individuals who have HH go through a gradual phase of asymptomatic iron loading into a symptomatic phase, ending with irreversible organ damage [6]. People who have HH absorb only a few milligrams of iron each day in excess of need; therefore, clinical manifestations occur only after 40 years of age when body stores of iron have reached 15 to 40 g [8,9,15]. Before the age of 30, symptoms are either absent or nonspecific [11,14]. The insidious nature of the disease results in an average time from onset of symptoms to diagnosis of 5 to 8 years [4]. Women are less likely to develop iron overload or they present with clinical expression later in life, likely because of blood loss through menstruation and pregnancy [5]. Phenotypic expression of HH involves a series of stages depicted in Table 1. Ideally, any screening would identify affected individuals before the third stage of the disease [1].

The primary storage site for iron is the liver, making it the first organ affected by HH. The gradual deposition of iron progresses to various other tissues, including the pancreas, joints, skin, heart, and pituitary gland. The patient develops hepatic fibrosis, diabetes mellitus, arthropathy, skin pigmentation changes, cardiomyopathy, and hypogonadotrophic hypogonadism [6].

The same HFE genotype may be expressed to different degrees in different individuals depending on environmental factors, such as age, sex,

Table 1
Stage, age of onset, and parenchymal iron storage in hereditary hemochromatosis

Stage	Age	Parenchymal iron storage
Iron overload without disease	0–20 y	0–5 g
Iron overload without disease	20–40 y	10–20 g
Iron overload with organ damage	>40 y	>20 g

diet, hepatitis C infection, iron loss through blood donation and menstruation, and the use of supplemental iron or vitamin C [5,6,15]. Ingestion of excessive alcohol is a major modifier of the expression of HH. Individuals who drink 60 g or more of alcohol per day are approximately nine times more likely to develop cirrhosis than those who drink less than 60 g per day.

Signs and symptoms

Most patients who have the HFE mutation remain asymptomatic with less than 1% of C282Y homozygotes developing frank clinical hemochromatosis [17]. H63D homozygotes or C282Y or H63D heterozygotes are usually phenotypically normal or have only mild iron overload. The S65C mutation is implicated in milder forms of HH [11].

HH is most frequently discovered incidentally or through the evaluation of abdominal pain, joint pain, or weakness [4]. Chronic fatigue, weakness, abdominal pain, joint and muscle pain, decreased libido, lethargy, and hepatomegaly are early clinical symptoms. The nonspecific nature of these symptoms, however, frequently results in a delayed diagnosis [9]. Fatigue, arthralgias, and impotence are the most common symptoms of the disorder. The classic presentation of HH is termed "bronze diabetes" and involves the triad of diabetes mellitus, skin pigmentation changes, and hepatomegaly [15]. This presentation, however, is only present in 8% of patients [4]. The most common signs and symptoms of HH are listed in Box 1.

The risk for cirrhosis is 13 times greater in patients who have HH than in the general population and liver dysfunction is present in 75% to 95% of people who have symptoms at diagnosis [4,11]. Hepatomegaly remains one of the more common physical signs in hemochromatosis but may not be present in young, asymptomatic individuals. Cirrhotic patients who abuse alcohol

Box 1. Common signs and symptoms
of hereditary hemochromatosis

Fatigue
Abdominal pain
Impotence
Arthropathy
Pigmentation changes
Decreased libido
Amenorrhea
Depression
Hypothyroidism
Muscle pain
Weakness
Arthralgias
Congestive heart failure
Diabetes mellitus
Hypogonadism
Testicular atrophy
Early menopause
Weight loss
Stiff joints
Cirrhosis

are more likely to have abnormal liver enzymes. Liver involvement leads to right upper quadrant pain, hepatomegaly, and mild transaminase elevations (AST, ALT). Marked elevations in liver enzymes and elevated iron tests should suggest an alternate diagnosis, such as alcoholic liver disease, chronic viral hepatitis, or nonalcoholic steatohepatitis. The liver can accumulate vast quantities of iron within the hepatocytes initially without any obvious sequelae in clinical symptoms or abnormal liver biochemistry [7]. Deposition of excess iron in hepatic parenchymal cells increases oxidative stress and increases the risk for cirrhotic tissue undergoing malignant transformation [5].

Iron deposition in the pancreas results in insulin resistance and subsequent beta cell failure in 80% of affected individuals [5]. Diabetes mellitus is present in approximately half of all patients at the time of HH diagnosis and the risk for developing diabetes is seven times higher in patients who have HH than in unaffected individuals [4].

Iron deposition within the joints may cause an inflammatory arthritis that is not related to the degree of iron overload. Joint disease develops in as many as 50% of patients who have HH, with arthropathy being present in 20% to 25% of patients. It does not improve after iron depletion.

The arthropathy of HH resembles osteoarthritis and is characterized by chondrocalcinosis from calcium pyrophosphate deposition and from deposition of hemosiderin in synovium [3]. The most commonly and most severely affected joints are those of the hand, particularly the second and third metacarpophalangeal joints. Progressive polyarthritis may involve the knees, wrists, and hip [5,11].

Deposition of iron in the pituitary leads to impaired gonadotropin release resulting in loss of sex drive, erectile dysfunction, impotence, and testicular atrophy in men, and amenorrhea or early menopause in women [5]. HH is considered responsible for sexual dysfunction in 10% to 40% of homozygous men [31].

The risk for cardiomyopathy is 306 times greater in patients who have HH than in those who do not have the disease [4]. Congestive heart failure is the presenting problem in approximately 10% of HH cases and up to one third of patients who have HH present with cardiac morbidity, especially a dilated cardiomyopathy caused by iron deposition in the myocardium. This cardiomyopathy results in a reduced ejection fraction and progresses to congestive heart failure with cardiac dysrhythmias [3]. Definitive diagnosis is commonly made with direct myocardial biopsy. Cardiac dysrhythmias and cardiomyopathy are the most common causes of sudden death in iron overload states and the risk for these complications can increase during rapid mobilization of iron [1]. C282Y carriers may have an increased risk for acute myocardial infarction and cardiovascular death [10].

Diagnostic testing

A case definition for HH has not been agreed on by experts [7]. Recently, increased emphasis has been placed on early detection of hemochromatosis, shifting the definition and diagnosis to earlier stages of the disease. This change has resulted in differing views on the best diagnostic methods and the essential components of the diagnostic evaluation [8].

At this time, the Centers for Disease Control does not recommend population-wide screening because of the uncertainty regarding how many individuals who have HFE mutations will develop clinically significant disease. To promote screening within the primary care setting, one must demonstrate that the disease is common, the burden is substantial, the treatment is efficacious, the screening tests are accurate, the screening is effective, and the benefits of screening outweigh the risks. The prevalence of HH within a primary care setting is 0.18% to 0.59% [19].

Symptomatic patients should be targeted for HH evaluation. This group includes individuals who have unexplained manifestations of liver disease or a presumably known cause of liver disease with abnormality of one or more indirect serum iron markers; type 2 diabetes mellitus, particularly with hepatomegaly; elevated liver enzymes; atypical cardiac disease; early-onset sexual dysfunction; or early-onset atypical arthropathy, cardiac disease, or male sexual dysfunction. Asymptomatic patients who should be targeted for HH evaluation include first-degree relatives of a confirmed case of HH, individuals who have abnormal serum iron markers discovered during routine testing, and individuals who have unexplained elevation of liver enzymes or the serendipitous finding of asymptomatic hepatomegaly or radiologic detection of enhanced CT attenuation of the liver [1].

The first phenotypic expression of HH is an elevation in serum transferrin saturation, representing the transport of excess iron from the intestine. As iron accumulates in tissues, the serum ferritin concentration increases in direct linear relation to total-body iron stores. The triad of increased serum iron, ferritin, and transferrin saturation characterizes classic HH [11]. Ninety-four percent of patients who have HH have one or more abnormalities in the serum iron level, serum ferritin level, or transferring saturation [4]. As serum iron markers have become more widely available, most patients who have HH are now identified while still asymptomatic and without evidence of hepatic fibrosis or cirrhosis [1]. It is crucial to diagnose hemochromatosis before cirrhosis develops because phlebotomy therapy can avert serious chronic disease and can even lead to normal life expectancy [10]. On average, however, three doctors and 9 years are required before a patient is correctly diagnosed [5].

The American Association for the Study of Liver Diseases (AASLD) recommends a three-step approach to the diagnosis of HH, including evaluating indirect serologic markers of iron stores, genotypic testing, and liver biopsy for hepatic iron concentration [1]. Iron stores are typically assessed using transferrin saturation and serum ferritin levels. Normally, serum iron-binding proteins in the plasma are one-third saturated and the reference range for percent saturation of transferrin is 20% to 50%. Transferrin saturation determines how much iron is bound to transferrin and is calculated using the following formula:

$$\text{Transferrin Saturation} = (\text{Serum Iron}/\text{TIBC}) \times 100 \text{ percent}$$

Individuals presenting for a routine medical assessment should have their transferrin saturation level measured because increasing transferrin saturation is the earliest biochemical abnormality in hereditary hemochromatosis and is attributed to increased intestinal iron absorption [19]. If the transferrin saturation is greater than 45% and verified by a second fasting sample, further investigation is warranted [10]. Overnight fasting avoids circadian or postprandial variations and eliminates 80% of false-positive transferrin saturation results [7]. When the fasting value exceeds 50% for women or 60% for men, transferrin saturation has a sensitivity of 0.92, a specificity of 0.93, and a positive predictive value of 86% for the diagnosis of HH. Lowering the cutoff transferrin saturation value to 45% increases sensitivity but reduces specificity and positive predictive value. The AASLD recommends a cutoff value of 45%, despite that it will also identify other groups with relatively minor degrees of secondary iron overload [1]. Transferrin saturation has a sensitivity of greater than 90% in most studies when a cutoff of 45% is considered and produces relatively few false-positive results [10,11]. The sensitivity of transferrin saturation is lower in population-based screening studies. Elevations of transferrin saturation have been associated with consumption of high doses of vitamin C, iron supplementation, and estrogen preparations and their use should be discontinued at least 24 hours before testing [5]. Unsaturated iron binding capacity has been proposed as a screening threshold with similar sensitivity and specificity to transferrin saturation but lower cost [7].

Within cells, iron is reversibly bound to ferritin [22]. Ferritin determines the level of iron stored in the body and correlates with hepatic iron content and development of cirrhosis. Diagnostically, increased sensitivity is achieved when the ferritin level and the transferrin saturation are considered jointly. When both laboratory tests are used simultaneously, the sensitivity is increased to 94% with a specificity of 86%, a positive predictive value of 73%, and a negative predictive value of 97% [1,4]. Values consistent with iron overload include a ferritin level greater than 300 μg/L in men and greater than 200 μg/L in women [9]. A ferritin less than 1000 μg/L is not usually associated with cirrhosis.

Serum ferritin is an acute-phase reactant and elevations may be related to age; other underlying liver diseases, such as alcoholic liver disease, chronic viral hepatitis, or nonalcoholic steatohepatitis; or to infection, cancer, heart disease, metabolic disorders, HIV, and other inflammatory conditions [2,5,7]. As the ferritin increases, the risk for significant liver disease also increases [7]. Checking the C-reactive protein or the erythrocyte sedimentation rate can help to identify if the elevated ferritin is attributable to inflammation or iron overload [10].

Patients who have a transferrin saturation less than 45% and a normal ferritin require no further testing. Elevations of transferrin saturation and serum ferritin warrant genotypic testing, however. Individuals who have serum indicators of iron overload who demonstrate an HFE mutation require phlebotomy therapy. First-degree relatives of known HH individuals may proceed directly to genotypic testing regardless of the transferrin saturation or serum ferritin [1]. The use of DNA-based tests alone may fail to identify 20% to 40% of white patients and most African American patients who have clinical evidence of HH who lack the C282Y mutation. Presumably, other genetic mutations are responsible for some cases of non-HFE–associated HH [8].

Liver biopsy is useful to document cirrhosis if it is not evident from radiologic studies and to rule out significant iron overload when iron markers are equivocal or to investigate other possible causes of liver disease. Although less frequently, liver biopsy is still being used to assess the degree of iron overload and to make a confirmative diagnosis of cirrhosis attributable to iron overload. Liver biopsy has shifted from a major diagnostic tool to a method of estimating prognosis and concomitant disease [7]. It is often reserved for individuals who do not have a recognizable genotype or for those for whom there is a risk for significant liver fibrosis [6].

In individuals who are not likely to have significant hepatic injury, liver biopsy is not necessary. This group includes individuals less than 40 years of age who have no clinical evidence of liver disease and whose serum ferritin is less than 1000 μg/L. Liver biopsy should be offered to document the degree of fibrosis in all homozygotes who are older than 40 years of age and who

have an elevated serum ALT, have clinical evidence of liver disease, or have a serum ferritin greater than 1000 ng/mL. Liver biopsy and evaluation of hepatic iron content are also recommended in compound heterozygotes (C282Y/ H63D), C282Y heterozygotes, or non-HFE– mutated individuals who have indirect markers of iron overload [1,10].

The degree and cellular distribution of iron stores is best assessed using a Perls Prussian blue stain. Iron deposition in hepatic parenchymal cells, especially in the periportal hepatocytes, generally is much more prominent than in Kupffer cells [7,8,10,15]. The normal hepatic iron concentration is less than 1800 μg/g dry weight. Patients who have HH who are older than 40 years of age and have a hepatic iron concentration exceeding 10,000 μg/g dry weight are more likely to show fibrosis or cirrhosis [1].

The hepatic iron concentration divided by age in years is the hepatic iron index. The hepatic iron index is defined as micromoles of iron per gram of dry liver divided by age in years [4]. A hepatic iron index greater than 1.9 μmol/g per year of life effectively distinguishes homozygous hemochromatosis from heterozygotes and patients who have other forms of chronic liver disease [1,8]. Up to 15% of genotypic homozygotes for HH do not meet the previously defined value of 1.9 μmol/g per year, however, and it is no longer considered essential for diagnosis. Although a hepatic iron index less than 1.9 does not entirely exclude HH, a value greater than this indicates significant iron overload in the C282Y homozygote and in individuals who have certain forms of secondary iron overload [1].

Additional testing for iron overload is being evaluated. MRI can demonstrate moderate to severe iron overload of the liver and may be helpful in establishing the diagnosis of hemochromatosis [7]. Studies have shown that several MRI methods can be used to quantify iron deposition in liver and cardiac tissue [21].

Treatment

Early treatment of HH with phlebotomy is highly effective because it reduces body iron stores to normal, prevents morbidity, and promotes normal longevity [1,14,18]. The goal of therapy is to remove excess iron to prevent further organ damage. Although posttreatment liver biopsies are not routinely done, iron depletion therapy has resulted in stabilization or reversal of hepatic fibrosis [6,7,9]. Signs and symptoms, such as malaise, fatigue, altered skin pigmentation, abdominal pain, lethargy, cardiomyopathy, conduction disturbances, elevated liver enzymes, hepatomegaly, and infectious complications, improve in most patients who have phlebotomy. Arthralgias, arthropathy, cirrhosis, hepatocellular carcinoma, diabetes mellitus, hypothyroidism, arthropathy, hypogonadism, and impotence do not usually improve [1,4,9,15].

Management objectives for HH include early diagnosis to prevent organ damage and dysfunction due to tissue iron toxicity; screening and early detection of asymptomatic HH cases to reduce mortality; recognition and diagnosis of symptomatic cases of HH to minimize progression and complications of the disease; adequate treatment of HH to promote rapid, safe, and effective iron removal; and vigilant follow-up and maintenance treatment of all cases of HH [10].

Although phlebotomy is the standard treatment of HH, it has never been subjected to a randomized clinical trial, limiting our understanding of the natural history of untreated disease [7]. Treatment consists of the initial removal of one unit (350–450 mL) of blood containing 200 to 250 mg of iron once or twice per week with regular monitoring of hemoglobin or hematocrit and serum ferritin levels after each gram of iron removed [3,10]. Before the next therapeutic phlebotomy, the hematocrit should have returned to within 10 points of or no lower than 20% less than the starting value.

Transferrin saturation usually remains elevated until iron stores are depleted. Ferritin may initially fluctuate, but it will eventually begin to fall progressively with iron mobilization. Serum ferritin should be measured after every 10 to 12 phlebotomies in initial stages of treatment.

Depending on the degree of excess body iron stores, the patient may require more than 100 phlebotomies and 2 to 3 years to deplete iron stores to the desired endpoint. The goal of phlebotomy therapy is to obtain iron depletion with ferritin levels less than 50 µg/L and a transferrin saturation less than 50% [1,3,5,10]. Maintenance phlebotomy is performed three to four times yearly to maintain ferritin levels less than 50 to 200 µg/L [4,10]. As the ferritin level gets close to 50 µg/L it should be measured more closely to prevent overt iron deficiency. Levels less than 25 µg/L indicate iron deficiency and require a temporary hold on phlebotomies. Iron deficiency anemia should be avoided [1]. Once the goals have been achieved,

yearly measurements of transferrin saturation and serum ferritin are recommended [4]. For maintenance therapy, certain people require phlebotomy every month, whereas others may need phlebotomy only three to four times per year [1].

Secondary treatment of HH or treatment when iron overload and anemia are present involves iron chelation therapy with deferoxamine (Desferal) [2,5]. Iron chelation is a process in which chemicals bind to iron, making a water-soluble complex that can then be excreted by the kidneys [16,23]. Deferoxamine is given intravenously and can reduce iron stores by approximately 60 mg/d [5]. Although intravenous deferoxamine is an effective iron chelator, it lacks the complete efficacy of phlebotomy [23]. It is much more expensive, less convenient, and has more side effects than phlebotomy. Daily supplemental folic acid is sometimes recommended in patients receiving phlebotomy to aid in hemoglobin formation and prevent anemia [16].

Patient education

Patients should be advised to avoid oral iron therapy and iron-containing supplements, but there are no proven dietary restrictions [7]. Many experts recommend, however, that patients be instructed to limit their dietary intake by avoiding foods rich in iron, including liver, meat, egg yolks, legumes, dried fruits, green leafy vegetables, broccoli, greens, and molasses. Additionally they should avoid foods fortified with iron, such as breads and cereals. Tea consumption has been shown to decrease intestinal iron absorption [4,7,23]. Alcohol increases absorption of iron and accelerates liver damage so patients who have liver disease should avoid alcohol completely [16,23].

Pharmacologic doses of vitamin C facilitate iron absorption and accelerate mobilization of iron to a level that may saturate circulating transferrin resulting in a potential increase in pro-oxidant and free radical activity; therefore, supplemental vitamin C should be avoided in patients undergoing phlebotomy. Patients receiving iron chelators should not exceed 200 to 500 mg of vitamin C per day [1,16,23].

Genetic screening of first-degree relatives and phenotypic testing of clinical suspects is the current standard most widely accepted by health care providers. Family members homozygous for the C282Y mutation should have serum transferrin saturation, ferritin, and liver enzyme levels evaluated [4,10]. The HFE gene test is most useful for screening adult family members of an identified proband. Screening family members is critical because 25% of the siblings and 5% of the children of a proband have HH [15]. Siblings have the highest chance of carrying the gene and should be screened with the genetic test, transferrin saturation, and serum ferritin. Phenotypic expression of the disease can vary widely between siblings suggesting that environmental factors are contributory [7,32]. Universal, population-based screening continues to be debated because genetic discrimination remains a major concern [6,7]. The major concerns around population-based screening for HH have been uncertainty surrounding the natural history of untreated disease, informed consent, payment for testing, labeling and stigmatization among participants who may never develop the illness, genetic discrimination in the health and life insurance realm, and concern associated with genetic testing in the absence of qualified genetic counseling [16,17,33,34].

Prognosis

Although patients who are homozygous for C282Y are more likely to have elevated serum ferritin levels and transferrin saturation, there is currently no way of predicting which patients will progress to overt disease [17]. Using a transferrin saturation greater than 50 in men and greater than 45 in women and a ferritin level of greater than 300 in men and greater than 200 in women, up to 38% to 50% of C282Y homozygotes develop iron overload and 10% to 33% develop end-stage organ disease and potentially life-threatening complications [8,9,13]. Documented cirrhosis at diagnosis does confer a worse prognosis with an adjusted relative risk for death of 5.5.

Hepatocellular carcinoma has been described in 18.5% of cirrhotic patients who have HH and accounts for approximately 30% of all deaths in HH. Individuals who have cirrhosis have an incidence of hepatoma 200 to 219 times higher than the general population [4,6,7]. Other complications of cirrhosis (eg, diabetes mellitus and cardiomyopathy) account for an additional 20% [1,7]. The risk for hepatocellular carcinoma is present even in patients who do not have cirrhosis despite iron depletion. It is possible that iron may have a direct mitogenic effect on the liver because of chronic stimulation of hepatocyte proliferation [6]. Life expectancy is reduced by 5 years on average [4]. Patients transplanted for HH have a poorer average survival after transplantation, often because of sepsis or cardiac events [2,7].

In chronic HCV infection, HFE mutations have been associated with increased iron deposition and accelerated thrombosis. Hepatitis C may directly modulate iron uptake into hepatocytes by increased expression of a second transferrin receptor [6].

Additionally, excessive hepatic iron concentration resulting from HH may decrease the effectiveness of interferon therapy for viral hepatitis [8].

Patients who have HH are susceptible to infections that are not commonly observed in unaffected individuals. These infections include *Yersinia* bacteremia, liver abscesses, *Listeria* meningitis, and endocarditis [29]. Raw shellfish should be avoided because patients who have HH are susceptible to infections caused by certain bacteria common in uncooked shellfish [23].

Summary

In summary, hereditary hemochromatosis is an autosomal recessive genetic disorder most frequently related to mutations on the HFE gene resulting in the substitution of the expected amino acids. The disease is most common in whites of northern European descent.

Individuals who have HH have increased total body iron stores that accumulate slowly over decades. The excess iron is deposited in the parenchyma of various organs, especially the liver, pancreas, heart, and endocrine glands, which results in end-organ disease and the development of cirrhosis, diabetes, cardiomyopathy, hypothyroidism, and impotence.

Diagnosis of phenotypically expressed HH relies on detection of elevated iron absorption and storage reflected by an elevated transferrin saturation and serum ferritin level. Patients who have elevated iron studies should have genetic testing for the HFE mutation.

Treatment is aimed at prevention of end-organ damage and involves therapeutic phlebotomies one to two times weekly until the patient has reached a state of iron deficiency. Treatment continues as needed to maintain the desired ferritin level. When treatment is initiated before the development of end-organ damage, the individual's life span is equal to those who do not have HH.

References

[1] Tivall AS. Diagnosis and management of hemochromatosis. Hepatology 2001;33(5):1321–8.

[2] Whittington CA, Kowdley KV. Review article: haemochromatosis. Aliment Pharmacol Ther 2002; 16:1963–75.

[3] Franchini M, Veneri D. Hereditary hemochromatosis. Hematology 2005;10(2):145–9.

[4] Little DR. Hemochromatosis: diagnosis and management. Am Fam Physician 1996;53(8):2623–8.

[5] Meeker JA, Miller SM. Hereditary hemochromatosis. MLO-Online 1996. p 10–8. Available at: www.mlo-online.com. Accessed September 16, 2007.

[6] Griffiths WJH. Review article: the genetic basis of haemochromatosis. Aliment Pharmacol Ther 2007; 26:331–42.

[7] Adams PC. Review article: the modern diagnosis and management of haemochromatosis. Aliment Pharmacol Ther 2006;23:1681–91.

[8] Powell LW, George DK, McDonnell SM, et al. Diagnosis of hemochromatosis. Ann Intern Med 1998;129(11):925–31.

[9] Whitlock EP, Garlitz BA, Harris EL, et al. Screening for hereditary hemochromatosis: a systematic review for the U.S. Preventive Services Task Force. Ann Intern Med 2006;145(3):209–23.

[10] Powell LW. Hereditary hemochromatosis and iron overload diseases. J Gastroenterol Hepatol 2002; 17:S191–5.

[11] Franchini M, Veneri D. Recent advances in hereditary hemochromatosis. Ann Hematol 2005;84:347–52.

[12] Distante S, Robson KJH, Graham-Campbell J, et al. Origin and spread of the HFE-C282Y haemochromatosis mutation. Hum Genet 2004;115:269–79.

[13] Anderson GJ, Ramm GA, Subramaniam VN, et al. Genetic disorders in gastroenterology and hepatology: HFE gene and hemochromatosis. J Gastroenterol Hepatol 2004;19:712.

[14] Rossi E, Henderson S, Chin CY, et al. Hepatobiliary diseases: genotyping as a diagnostic aid in genetic haemochromatosis. J Gastroenterol Hepatol 1999; 14:427–30.

[15] Brandhagen DJ, Fairbanks VE, Baldus W. Recognition and management of hereditary hemochromatosis. Am Fam Physician 2002;65(5):853–60.

[16] Dolbey CH. Hemochromatosis: a review. Clin J Oncol Nurs 2001;5(6):257–60.

[17] Qaseem A, Aronson M, Fitterman N, et al. Screening for hereditary hemochromatosis: a clinical practice guideline from the American College of Physicians. Ann Intern Med 2005;143:517–21.

[18] Matas M, Guiz P, Castro JA, et al. Prevalence of HFE C282Y and H63D in Jewish populations and clinical implication of H63D homozygosity. Clin Genet 2006;69:155–62.

[19] Schmitt B, Golub RM, Green R. Screening primary care patients for hereditary hemochromatosis with transferrin saturation and serum ferritin level: systematic review for the American College of Physicians. Ann Intern Med 2005; 143(7):522–36.

[20] Cardoso CS, de Sousa M. HFE, the MHC and hemochromatosis: paradigm for an extended function for MHC class I. Tissue Antigens 2003; 61:263–75.

[21] Ptasek LM, Price ET, Hu MY, et al. Early diagnosis of hemochromatosis-related cardiomyopathy with magnetic resonance imaging. J Cardiovasc Magn Reson 2005;7:689–92.

[22] Donovan A, Andrews NC. The molecular regulation of iron metabolism. Hematol J 2004;5:373–80.

[23] De Sevo MR. Would you suspect this genetic disorder? RN 2005;68(3):47–50.

[24] Distante S. Genetic predisposition to iron overload: prevalence and phenotypic expression of hemochromatosis-associated HFE-C282Y gene mutation. Scand J Clin Lab Invest 2006;66: 83–100.

[25] Barton JC, Acton RT, Lovato L, et al. Initial screening transferrin saturation values, serum ferritin concentrations, and HFE genotypes in Native Americans and whites in the hemochromatosis and Iron Overload Screening Study. Clin Genet 2006; 69:48–57.

[26] Yunker LM, Parboosingh JS, Conradson HE, et al. The effect of iron status on vascular health. Vasc Med 2006;11:85–91.

[27] Deicher R, Horl WH. New insights into the regulation of iron homeostasis. Eur J Clin Invest 2006;36:301–9.

[28] Pietrangelo A. Hereditary hemochromatosis. Annu Rev Nutr 2006;26:251–70.

[29] Luft FC. Hepcidin comes to the rescue. J Mol Med 2004;82:345–7.

[30] Anderson GJ, Frazer DM. Iron metabolism meets signal transduction. Nat Genet 2006;38(5):503–4.

[31] Van deursen C, Delaere K, Tenkate J. Hemochromatosis and sexual dysfunction. Int J Impot Res 2003;15:430–2.

[32] Beutler E. Editorial: natural history of hemochromatosis. Mayo Clin Proc 2004;79(3):305–6.

[33] Adams PC. Screening for haemochromatosis—producing or preventing illness? Lancet 2005;366: 269–71.

[34] U.S. Preventive Services Task Force. Screening for hemochromatosis: recommendation statement. Ann Intern Med 2006;145(3):204–8.

ELSEVIER
SAUNDERS

Crit Care Nurs Clin N Am 20 (2008) 203–212

CRITICAL CARE
NURSING CLINICS
OF NORTH AMERICA

Genes and Acute Neurologic Disease and Injury: A Primer for the Neurologic Intensive Care Nurse

Sheila A. Alexander, RN, PhD*, Michael Beach, MSN, ACNP-BC

Department of Acute and Tertiary Care, School of Nursing, University of Pittsburgh, 336 Victoria Building, 3500 Victoria Street, Pittsburgh, PA 15261, USA

The completion of sequencing of the human genome and the explosion of clinical research and application of genetic data to the clinical arena have not bypassed the neuroscience community. Although treatments for many neurologic diseases and injuries are supportive in nature, results of research driven by findings from the human genome project are promising. There is little research exploring associations between genes and neurologic disease or injury for patients in the intensive care setting. There is some preclinical work exploring pathways involved in neurologic disease and injury and acute response of the central nervous system to disease and injury. As more of this work is tested in humans, knowledge of pathways influencing response will help us to improve outcomes for these patients. The pathways involved in neurologic response to disease and injury are influenced by an individual's genetic makeup. This article serves to educate critical care nurses of the current state of the science of genetic influences on acute neurologic disease and injury commonly seen by nurses in the neurologic intensive care unit.

Genetic influences on neurologic disease development

There are many neurologic diseases with a known genetic cause, such as Huntington chorea and muscular dystrophy, and even more with a known pattern of inheritance for which no causative gene has yet been identified. Additionally,

recent research is identifying genes that influence pathways of many common neurologic diseases. Some of these neurologic diseases with a potential genetic influence are seen in ICUs. There is also much research being done to determine pathways involved in survival in more common neurologic illness and injury. Research exploring the development of multiple sclerosis (MS), stroke, and traumatic brain injury (TBI) has been included in this review.

Multiple sclerosis

MS is an inflammatory disease affecting the central nervous system and is hallmarked by demyelination and axonal loss from abnormal immune response. The disease clusters in families, suggesting a genetic contribution to its development. Although no single gene responsible for MS has been identified, research exploring genetic influences on development of MS and response to treatment is changing the face of health care for the patient who has MS. Some researchers have explored the association between single genes and MS without success. For instance, Lundmark and colleagues [1] explored the role of the promoter polymorphisms in the myeloperoxidase (MPO) gene in MS. MPO is an enzyme released by neutrophils during the inflammatory response that causes tissue damage and is therefore believed to be a good candidate gene for predicting MS risk. Although these researchers had a large sample size (871 patients who had MS and 532 healthy controls), they found no significant association with risk for MS. Heggarty and associates [2] have investigated the role of Cytotoxic T-lymphocyte-associated protein 4 (CTLA4) polymorphisms in a population

---

* Corresponding author.

E-mail address: salexand@pitt.edu (S.A. Alexander).

of relapsing-remitting and primary-progressive MS patients. A single nucleotide polymorphism (SNP) in exon 1 (+49) was associated with the relapsing-remitting population in a dose–response manner; having two copies of the SNP was more highly associated with the disease (odds ratio [OR] = 1.70, 95% CI = 1.11–2.61, $P = .015$) than having one copy of the SNP (OR = 1.36, 95% CI = 1.11–1.81, $P = .038$). In the primary-progressive MS population, overall allele distribution of the 3′UTR (AT(n)) microsatellite was different from the healthy controls The researchers found no association with the promoter polymorphism or intergenic CT60 SNPs in either of the MS cohorts. The findings of this study highlight variation in the CTLA4 +49 A/G and 3′UTR as genes that may modify the expression of MS.

Searching for a single gene responsible for development of MS is costly and difficult because it is likely a disease process with a multifactorial focus, meaning that a combination of genes interact with one another and with environmental influences to produce the phenotype. As such, and with development of newer technologies, research has turned to exploring the entire genome of patients who have MS. The International Multiple Sclerosis Genetics Consortium, a group with the purpose of identifying genes influencing risk for developing MS, has recently made some interesting findings. Using DNA microarray technology on samples from 931 family trios (an affected child and both biologic parents) with an additional 609 family trios and 789 control subjects used for replication they were able to estimate significance of various genes and the risk for MS. In the family trios, they found 49 SNPs were associated with MS ($P < 1 \times 10[-4]$), of which 38 were considered for second-stage analysis. Comparison between the MS case subjects (affected individual from the family trio) and the control subjects identified 32 additional SNPs ($P < .001$) associated with MS. When the criteria for significance were widened to include SNPs with P values less than .01 (rather than < .001), an additional 40 SNPs were identified. A total of 110 SNPs were then selected for the second-stage analysis. In this second-stage analysis, several influential genes were identified. In particular, two SNPs within the interleukin-2 receptor alpha gene (IL2RA) ($P = 2.96 \times 10[-8]$) and one SNP in the interleukin-7 receptor alpha gene (IL7RA) ($P = 2.94 \times 10[-7]$) were strongly associated with the MS cohort. The also found multiple SNPs in the human leukocyte antigen–DRA

locus ($P = 8.94 \times 10[-81]$) were significantly associated with MS [3].

Additional work exploring genetic response to pharmacologic treatment of MS has been promising. Because there is variability in patient response to medications for MS and the treatment requires long-term adherence and monitoring, a focus of research in MS is on genetic-based optimization of drug regimens. Grossman and colleagues [4] set out to identify a genetic marker to predict response to glatiramer acetate (Copaxone) immunotherapy, a common treatment of relapsing MS. They genotyped HLA DRB1*1501 and 61 SNPs within 27 candidate genes in samples from subjects enrolled in two glatiramer acetate clinical trials. They were able to analyze the influences of individual SNPs and haplotypes in drug-treated versus placebo-treated groups, a strong study design. Significant associations were found between glatiramer acetate response and a T cell receptor β variant SNP (OR = 6.85) in both cohorts, and a cathepsin S gene (OR = 11.59; $P = .049$) in one cohort. Additionally, in the glatiramer acetate-treated group (and not the placebo group), trends suggested possible associations between drug response and SNPs in other genes, including MBP, CD86, FAS, IL1R1, and IL12RB2. The authors suggest these genes are involved in the mechanism by which glatiramer acetate works.

Stroke

Stroke, the death of brain tissue from various sources, is a major cause of death and disability in the United States. The cost of lifetime care to stroke patients in the United States was estimated to be greater than $40 billion in 1990 [5]. With the increasing costs of health care and the increase in average age of Americans, the total anticipated cost of stroke care is increasing. The anticipation of this huge financial and human burden has led to an increase in the amount of research being done to explore potential risk factors and treatments to improve outcome from stroke. Currently therapies are limited, with the primary focus being on supporting systems while the brain heals itself. Knowledge from the human genome project is being used to determine pathways of damage after stroke and therapeutics are sure to follow. Pathways of injury after stroke are well defined. A decrease in oxygen and nutrient delivery to brain tissue leads to hypoxia and eventually ischemia. Ischemia leads to neuronal, astrocytic, and microglial cell death. This cell death leads to impairment in physical, cognitive, and emotional function. There are many pathways involved in the evolution of stroke and subsequent cell death. Current research is focused on further definition of pathways and points at which we can safely intervene to improve cell survival and thereby outcomes.

Ischemic stroke

Matarin and associates [6] attempted a comparison genome-wide analysis of results from a cohort of 249 subjects who had ischemic stroke and 268 subjects who did not have stroke. They assayed more than 40,000 SNPs. They found no single locus explaining a large effect on ischemic stroke. They made their data public earlier this year; however, no further analysis of this cohort data has been published.

Lalouschek and colleagues [7] explored the prevalence of 60 polymorphisms in 35 genes in 450 white patients who had acute stroke or transient ischemic attack and 817 healthy control individuals. They found that frequencies of all examined polymorphisms were similar in the two populations and there was no significant influence of these genes on risk for stroke. Research exploring SNPs of genes will likely be more fruitful if genes with products involved in pathways influencing stroke are targeted.

Genetics contribute significantly to a person's risk for an ischemic stroke. Ischemic strokes are the most common cerebral vascular accident (CVA). Intimal-medial wall thickness (IMT) of the carotid arteries is a significant measure of subclinical arthrosclerosis and a predictor of ischemic stroke. In a study by Jerrard-Dunne and colleagues [8], 5400 people were examined for a parental history of CVA or myocardial infarction and increased IMT. It was found that IMT has a significant familial component that is independent of other risk factors. Humphries reviewed several studies and articles that examined the genetic influences on various enzymes that exhibit influences on IMT [9].

Matrix metalloproteinase 3 (MMP3) regulates vascular remodeling through its effect on the accumulation of extracellular matrix during tissue injury. It is regulated at the transcription phase and is affected by such factors as growth factors and cytokines. Although no firm link to a particular gene has been found, there is evidence that IMT may be linked to genes that influence matrix distribution through MMP3. Inheritability

estimates range from 30% to 40%. There is a common variant within the alleles upstream from the start of transcription. One was found to have five adenosine nucleotides (5A) and another had 6 (6A). Site 5A was found to have significantly more activity than 6A, which would indicate that those people who had the 5A genetic variation would have a higher MMP3 concentration in the arterial walls. Because this would increase proteolytic activity, there would be less buildup of the atherosclerotic plaques. People who have the 6A marker are therefore at higher risk for an ischemic CVA and possibly myocardial infarction.

Ischemic stroke initiates an inflammatory response in the central nervous system. Interleukin (IL)–6 plays an important role in the inflammatory process, including the production of C-reactive protein. The inflammatory process has been associated with endothelial dysfunction, including adhesion molecule release. Humphries' analysis speculates that it may be pivotal in the inflammatory pathogenesis of arterial disease, including IMT. IL-6 is a glycoprotein located on chromosome 7p21 and is regulated through various transcription factor binding sites. For example, glucocorticoid suppression occurs at the glucocorticoid binding site. With some variation, the 174G allele is most associated in various studies with the regulation of IL-6. Variation in the IL-6 gene has been explored as a potential predictor of stroke, and Greisenegger and associates found that the −174 G/C polymorphism is associated with more severe ischemic stroke [10]. Lee and associates [11] explored the prevalence of genes with cytokine products, including IL-6, tumor necrosis factor (TNF)–α, TNF-β, IL-1β, IL-10, and IL-1Rα in 105 subjects who had ischemic stroke and 389 control subjects. They found none of these genes independently associated with stroke, but the IL-6 −174 CC genotype was significantly lower in stroke patients who did not have a history of hypertension. Worrall and colleagues [12] performed an association study exploring the variable number of tandem repeats in the IL1RN gene in North Americans. The study incorporated data from three studies—one using sibling pairs with history of stroke and two cohorts of subjects and unrelated controls. They found that after adjustment for age, sex, and stroke risk factors, allele 2 of IL1RN gene was associated with ischemic stroke development (OR 2.8, 95% CI 1.29–6.11, $P = .03$) for white participants but there was no association for nonwhite participants. Others have found similar results for IL-1Rα and TNF-α (but not IL-1β) polymorphisms in other populations of both genders [11,13–17]. A study of Japanese patients who had stroke found a higher frequency of variant haplotypes in the C-reactive protein gene when compared with controls [18].

Cyclooxygenase-2, a pro-atherogenic factor produced during inflammation, has been explored for its potential influences on stroke risk. Colaizzo and associates [19] explored the association between the G/C −765, a SNP within the COX-2 promoter region, in 110 patients who had ischemic stroke and 394 controls. Being homozygous for the CC allele was found to be an independent predictor of decreased risk for ischemic stroke after controlling for confounding variables.

Homocysteine is an enzyme that has been associated with increased risk for cardiovascular disease. The gene encoding 5,10-methylenetetrahydrofolate reductase (MTHFRC677T) is associated with hyperhomocysteinemia. Cronin and associates performed a meta-analysis of studies reporting frequencies of MTHFR 677 alleles in patients who had stroke and transient ischemic attack. In a population of 14,870 subjects, they found the pooled estimated risk for stroke or transient ischemic attack associated with the variant allele (T) was elevated with each copy of the variant allele (OR = 1.17, 95% CI = 1.09–1.26 for at least one T; OR = 1.37, 95% CI = 1.15–1.64 for TT genotype) [20].

Stroke susceptibility was previously mapped to chromosome 5q12 [21]. Further work mapped the locus and found the gene encoding phosphodiesterase 4D (PDE4D) is associated with ischemic stroke [22]. Phosphodiesterase 4D is an enzyme that metabolizes cyclic AMP and is found in inflammatory and immune cells. Association analysis of SNPs in the PDE4D gene in an Icelandic stroke cohort demonstrated genetic association between six SNPs in the 5′ region of PDE4D and ischemic stroke [12]. These findings have been repeated in other populations. Fidani and associates [23] explored the association of PDE4D gene G0 haplotype and ischemic stroke in a Greek population. They considered the role of an SNP (SNP45) and microsatellite marker (AC008818-1) in a cohort of patients and control subjects and found that one allele (148) was associated with an increased risk for stroke, whereas another allele (144) had a protective effect. Others have found similar results [24,25].

Lipid content can also influence stroke development by increasing atherosclerotic plaque development. Genetic influences play an important role in the management of lipids by the body. Genes involved in lipid storage, transport, and metabolism have been explored in relation to ischemic stroke [26]. Hepatic lipase is an enzyme that plays a particularly important role in the control of lipoproteins. It is responsible for lipolysis of very low-density lipoprotein and the conversion of high-density lipid 2 into high-density lipid 3, a smaller lipoprotein. High levels of hepatic lipase are associated with increases in the number of small dense low-density lipids and an increased risk for atherosclerosis and vascular events. A strong allele association has been shown between the 480C allele and low hepatic lipase levels. There are conflicting studies on this and there is no published study that specifically examines the relationship between hepatic lipase and cerebrovascular accidents. Lymphotoxin-α gene 252G allelic variant promotes atherosclerotic plaque growth. The SNP was more common in 353 patients who had stroke than in 1890 healthy controls (13.9 versus 7.2%, $P < .025$) [27]. A study of Chinese subjects who had stroke (n = 1825) and controls (n = 1817) explored pentanucleotide TTTTA repeat (PNTR) polymorphism of the apolipoprotein (apo) a gene and stroke subtypes. Low-number repeats (<16 in both alleles) of apo(a) PNTR were associated with atherothrombotic (OR = 1.41, 95% CI = 1.04–1.91) and hemorrhagic stroke (OR = 1.62, 95% CI = 1.09–2.37). Similar work in a Japanese population (177 patients who had stroke, 177 healthy controls) has found that variants in the lipoprotein lipase gene, another gene with a role in lipid metabolism, are associated with stroke risk. The Ser4447Stop mutation was associated with increased risk for stroke (0.107 versus 0.158 for healthy controls, $P = .035$) [28].

Humphries, in his review, also found a positive relationship between apolipoprotein E (APOE) and an increase in IMT. The common variations of the gene responsible for the production of APOE, e2, e3, and e4 isoforms act as predictors of lipid concentrations. Several studies also indicate a connection between the e4 allele and a higher IMT. Several studies and a meta-analysis by McCarron have indicated an association between stroke and the e4 allele.

Because of the relationship between cardiovascular and cerebrovascular health, genes influencing the cardiovascular system are prime candidates for study as potential predictors of stroke. As such, genes influencing the renin-angiotensin-aldosterone system have been considered for their potential to predict stroke. A study of 215 subjects who had ischemic stroke and 236 controls considered genes of the renin-angiotensin-aldosterone system (M235T polymorphism of angiotensinogen gene, D/I polymorphic site of the ACE gene; −T344C promoter polymorphism in the aldosterone synthase gene, and the A1166C polymorphism in the angiotensin II type I receptor gene). Only one gene was associated with stroke, the C1166/AT1 gene variant (OR = 1.5, 95% CI = 1.1–2.2, P = .024) [29]. Although not included in the meta-analysis by Casas and colleagues, there have not been further studies confirming this relationship.

Genes involved in thrombosis regulation and inflammatory response, specifically the thrombomodulin Ala455Val polymorphism, have been associated with increased risk for stroke. In another study using the Stroke Prevention in Young Women Study data, the AA genotype (compared with AV and VV genotypes) was found to be significantly associated with stroke after controlling for age, race, cigarette smoking, hypertension, and diabetes (OR = 1.9, 95% 2CI = 1.1–3.3) [30]. Another study explored genotypes of platelet glycoprotein IIb/IIIa, a platelet adhesion membrane receptor, with ischemic stroke. The PLA2 (versus PLA1) allele was present about twice as often in individuals who had stroke (23.3% versus 11.7% in controls, $P < .0005$) [31]. Variant polymorphisms in the fibrinolytic gene have also been shown to be associated with myocardial infarction; however, they are not associated with increased risk for ischemic stroke [32].

Because of the lack of oxygen and then reperfusion associated with stroke, oxidative stress occurs after stroke and can cause additional damage. Plasma glutathione is an antioxidant enzyme that serves to protect tissue by reducing reactive oxygen species. There is some promise in research exploring influence of polymorphisms in the promoter region of the plasma glutathione peroxidase (GPx-3) gene and ischemic stroke. This study used 123 young adults who had idiopathic arterial ischemic stroke and 123 age- and gender-matched healthy controls. They found two main haplotypes (H1 and H2) of eight polymorphisms in the promoter region present in this population and the H2 haplotype was overrepresented, suggesting a potential role for stroke development. It was associated with risk for acute ischemic stroke in young adults (OR = 2.07, 95% CI = 1.03–4.47, P = .034) and children (OR = 2.13, 95% CI = 1.23–4.90, P = .027). Transcriptional activity of the H2 haplotype was lower than that of the H1 haplotype. The authors hypothesize the haplotype reduces the gene's transcriptional activity, thereby compromising gene expression and plasma antioxidant and antithrombotic activities [33]. Nitric oxide (NO), a known free radical, has known vasodilatory effects and the gene driving its production in endothelial cells (eNOS) has also been explored as a possible risk factor for stroke. In a study using the Stroke Prevention in Young Women data, a case control study, eNOS polymorphisms were explored in 110 ischemic stroke cases and 206 case controls (all female) 15 to 44 years old. This study found two SNPs in the eNOS promoter region (G-922A and −T786A) were associated with ischemic strokes, but only in the black women [34,35].

Atrial natriuretic peptide (ANP) is a hormone that regulates blood pressure by altering fluid and sodium balance. Because hypertension has been associated with increased risk for stroke, polymorphisms of the ANP gene have also been associated with increased risk for ischemic stroke. A study from Italy involving 206 stroke subjects and 236 controls found presence of the ANP/TC2238 variant associated with increased risk for stroke (OR = 3.8, 95% CI = 1.4–10.9). When combined with the allelic variant of the NPRA gene (ANP receptor), the two genes together were associated with an even higher risk (OR = 5.5, 95% CI = 1.5–19.4) [36].

There are multiple physiologic pathways involved in stroke. As such, there are likely many genes affecting stroke risk at various points along these pathways. Environmental factors are also known to influence stroke risk. With multiple genetic and environmental factors influencing multiple pathways that influence overall stroke risk, finding the contribution of one single gene to stroke risk is difficult. It requires well-designed prospective studies and large sample sizes. The relationship between candidate genes and ischemic stroke is ideal for meta-analysis. A meta-analysis of candidate gene studies in ischemic stroke published in 2004 by Casas and associates [37] attempted to identify single genes significantly associated with ischemic stroke risk. The authors included case-control studies published in English with neuroimaging evidence of diagnosis. They included studies with white adult populations only. The authors pooled the data from 120 studies and found significant associations with ischemic stroke for the following genes: factor V Leiden Arg506Gln (OR = 1.33, 95% CI = 1.12–1.58, n = 4588), methylenetetrahydrofolate reductase C677T (OR = 1.24, 95% CI = 1.08–1.42, n = 3387), prothrombin G20210A (OR = 1.44, 95% CI = 1.11–1.86, n = 3028), and angiotensin-converting enzyme insertion/deletion (OR = 1.21, 95% CI = 1.08–1.35, n = 2990). They found no significant association between ischemic stroke and the following genes: factor XIII, apolipoprotein E, and human platelet antigen type 1. Other studies have validated the significant associations of these genes in other populations [38–40]. In some populations, different results have been found. For instance, in a meta-analysis, McCarron and associates found the APOE e4 allele was present in higher frequency in stroke patients (n = 926) when compared with age- and sex-matched controls (n = 890) (OR = 1.73, 95% CI = 1.34–2.23, $P < .001$) [41]. Additional work in other populations has also supported these findings [42,43]. It is clear that there is a genetic component to stroke; however, it is likely a compilation of the effects of variations in multiple genes interacting with the environment that ultimately leads to pathophysiology leading to stroke.

The development of therapies to improve outcome has been limited, but in recent years there has been some improvement primarily because of the administration of tissue plasminogen activator to break up clots blocking the cerebral vasculature. There has been significant work in recent years defining genetic differences in recovery from ischemic stroke. Pathways leading to damage from ischemia after stroke are being clarified and many have genotypic influences. One such gene is poly-ADP ribose polymerase (PARP), a DNA repair enzyme that also mediates cell death by way of energy depletion. Oxidative stress after ischemia causes DNA damage, which activates PARP-1. PARP-1 activation leads to a chain of secondary events that impact cell survival. Although PARP-1 activation sets into motion a cascade that promotes cellular survival, excessive PARP-1 activation leads to energy depletion and cell death [44]. A PARP-1 inhibitor has shown effectiveness in reducing infarct volume in animal models of ischemic stroke [45]. Although no PARP-1 inhibitors are currently approved and available for use in humans, clinical trials are ongoing to move one PARP-1 inhibitor into the clinical arena.

Intracerebral hemorrhage

Several individual genes have also been explored as potential risk factors for hemorrhagic stroke. Genes involved in the coagulation cascade and development of hypertension are often considered because of the physiologic role of their gene products. Factor XIII is an enzyme involved in the clotting cascade. Factor XIII-A Val34Leu polymorphism presence has been associated with intracerebral hemorrhage; in one study of 130 patients who had intracerebral hemorrhage (compared with 200 healthy controls) the variant allele was present more often than in the healthy control sample (n = 200) (33.8% versus 23.1%, $P = .009$) yet present less often in the ischemic stroke/transient ischemic attack sample (n = 240) (17.3% versus 24.2% in healthy controls, $P = .011$) [46].

Presence of the APOE e4 allele has also been implicated as a risk factor for intracerebral hemorrhage and subarachnoid hemorrhage (SAH) in many populations. One study by Kokubo and colleagues [47] found APOE e4 allele carriers had a 2.5-fold increased risk for SAH (OR = 2.4, 95% CI = 1.3–4.6) and 1.8-fold higher risk for intracerebral hemorrhage (OR = 1.8, 95% CI = 1.0–3.3).

Subarachnoid hemorrhage

SAH is a unique stroke subtype involving bleeding into the subarachnoid space around the brain. Cerebral aneurysm rupture is the most common cause of subarachnoid hemorrhage. Currently, only one gene has been associated with cerebral aneurysm formation. In a study of 76 subjects who had intracranial aneurysms and 93 control subjects, a variant allele in the promoter region of the matrix metalloproteinase-9 (MMP-9) gene was associated with increased transcription of this gene, which may influence aneurysm formation [48]. These results have not been verified by others.

Acute response to SAH is also being explored from a genetic viewpoint. Although no single gene has been identified as being responsible for the development of cerebral vasospasm, the most common cause of delayed secondary injury after SAH, many genes are currently being explored with promising results for potential future therapeutic use. NO is a strong vasodilator and is produced by both vasculature and neurons. Genotypic differences in the NO synthases (proteins that produce NO) result in varying levels of NO production and may influence vasomotor tone and therefore cerebral vasospasm. Currently endothelial NO synthase (eNOS) has been studied extensively. Khurana and associates (2004) [49] found that in 141 patients who had SAH, the eNOS gene intron-4 27-base pair variable number tandem repeat polymorphism (eNOS 27 VNTR) was associated with aneurysm rupture, and the eNOS gene promoter T-786C SNP was associated with cerebral vasospasm.

Plasminogen activator inhibitor-1 (PAI-1) is a major inhibitor of tissue plasminogen activator and hence fibrinolysis. Increased blood in the subarachnoid space after SAH has been associated with cerebral vasospasm, the primary cause of cerebral ischemia after SAH [50]. A study by Vergouwen and colleagues [51] explored PAI-1 promoter polymorphism SNPs in association with development of cerebral ischemia and other secondary injuries commonly occurring after SAH. They found that in 126 patients who had SAH, the 4G genotype was associated with increased cerebral ischemia and poor outcomes as compared with homozygotes for the 5G genotype.

In an effort to consider whether multiple target genes might interact to influence recovery from SAH, Ruigrok and associates [52] explored functional polymorphisms in APOE, insulinlike growth factor-1 (IGF-1), TNF-α, IL-1α, IL-1β, and IL-6 genes in relation to outcome in 167 patients who had SAH. They found that patients who had the IGF-1 variant had a lower risk for poor outcome (OR = 2.3, 95% CI = 0.2–1.0), whereas those who had the TNF-α variant had a higher risk for poor outcome (OR = 2.3, 95% CI = 1.0–5.4). None of the other polymorphisms were correlated with outcome.

Although primarily known for its lipid transport and metabolism capabilities, apoE has other functions, including ionic homeostasis [53–55], synaptic plasticity [56–58], and regeneration [59,60]. It has been explored as a potential influence on recovery from SAH. A meta-analysis of the existing literature (five studies) found that individuals who had the APOE4 allele had nearly threefold increased risk for developing delayed neurologic deterioration after SAH (OR = 2.558, 95% CI = 1.610–4.065) [61].

At this time there are no therapies for SAH based on genotype. There are also no genes with a strong enough association with aneurysm development to be used as a screening tool. The rapid rate at which technology is being developed for genetic and proteomic testing will lead to increased screening to identify individuals at risk for aneurysm development, SAH, cerebral vasospasm, and poor outcome after SAH.

Genetic influences on recovery from traumatic injury

Treatments for acute neurologic injuries, and particularly brain and spinal cord injuries, are limited and primarily supportive in nature. Currently there is much research exploring genetic influences on mechanisms involved in ischemia, necrosis, and apoptosis—all common occurrences after brain and spinal cord injury (SCI). Insight into mechanism of secondary injury will aid in the development of therapeutics aimed at limiting cell death after neurologic injuries and will also drive genetically based prognostic indicators and genetically based individualized care.

Traumatic brain injury

TBI is a well-described phenomenon with temporal changes in cerebral blood flow, amino acid release, inflammatory response, and cellular death pathways. The care provided to patients recovering from TBI varies based on severity of the injury, but is currently aimed at monitoring and preventing secondary injuries. Research in animal models suggests future treatments may improve outcomes by targeting cellular-level responses, increasing neuronal survival, and ultimately saving brain tissue.

Presence of the APOE e4 allele has been associated with poor outcome after TBI [62–65]. The role APOE plays in response to TBI is complex and likely involves multiple pathways. In one study by Kerr and associates [66], in 91 patients who had severe TBI (Glasgow coma score ≤8) those who had the APOE e4 allele had significantly higher levels of aspartate and lactate/pyruvate over the first 5 days after injury ($P < .001$) after controlling for potential covariates, suggesting altered metabolism. Another study found that in 54 subjects who had severe TBI (Glasgow coma score ≤8), those who had the APOE e4 allele had increased global cerebral blood flow ($P = .02$) after controlling for other potential covariates [67]. In a study of 89 subjects who had TBI, Teasdale and associates [65] found that subjects who had the APOE e4 allele had worse outcomes than those who did not have the APOE e4 allele 6 months after injury ($P = .06$). These findings have been verified by others [62–65].

Because there is a strong inflammatory response initiated after TBI, there has also been significant work exploring cytokines. TNF-α and ILs have suggested a potential role in response to TBI. In a study of 28 subjects who had severe TBI, mean cerebrospinal fluid IL-10 was elevated compared with control samples [68]. Although the current research is focused on proteins, the genes influencing cytokine production and metabolism will inform standards of care for this population. As the pathways influencing recovery from TBI are explored through a genetic lens additional therapies will be designed to influence different points along those pathways.

Spinal cord injury

SCI has been a challenge to clinicians. Neurons and glial cells are damaged and eventually die off, causing paresis and paralysis. A cascade of events following the injury leads to damage to tissues adjacent to the injury causing further damage, more cell death, and resultant loss of additional function. The injured spinal cord is not able to regenerate and deficits are generally permanent. There are currently no effective therapeutic options to improve function after SCI. There are some potential future therapeutics based on promising results from research in animal models. Transplantation of embryonic stem cells, which are able to differentiate into multiple cell types, has been explored in animal models of SCI. Embryonic stem cell–derived neural progenitor cells can differentiate into motor neurons in culture [69]. The environment within the central nervous system is not hospitable for stem cells to differentiate into neurons; rather, they become glial cells [70,71]. Although these studies have been in culture or animal models, research continues and the results are promising.

Summary

Neurologic illness and injury are extremely difficult to treat and few treatments have shown clinical efficacy. The knowledge gained during the genetic revolution has great potential to drive developments of therapeutics aimed at improving outcome from neurologic disease and injury. Many pathways influencing central nervous system response to injury have been identified in animal models and attempts are being made to verify the role of these pathways in human response to injury. Genetics influence all these pathways and may explain some of the variation in recovery seen in the acutely ill neurologic patient. Currently, most of the work exploring genetics and neurologic disease and injury relevant to critical care nurses is related to patients recovering from stroke. TBI is another area in which genetic influences on recovery have been explored, although few genes have been considered. Knowledge of pathways associated with neuronal survival (or death) helps researchers identify areas to intervene in those pathways to improve outcomes. As we learn more about mechanism of disease and injury and the role genetic response plays in recovery from neurologic diseases and injuries, individualized interventions will likely be developed and patient outcomes will improve. Certainly, this is an exciting time to be involved in care of the neurologically injured patient.

References

[1] Lundmark F, Salter H, Hillert J. An association study of two functional promoter polymorphisms in the myeloperoxidase (MPO) gene in multiple sclerosis. Mult Scler 2007;13:697–700.

[2] Heggarty S, Suppiah V, Silversides J, et al. CTLA4 gene polymorphisms and multiple sclerosis in Northern Ireland. J Neuroimmunol 2007;187–91.

[3] International Multiple Sclerosis Genetics Consortium, Hafler DA, Compston A, Sawcer S, et al. Risk alleles for multiple sclerosis identified by a genomewide study [see comment]. N Engl J Med 2007;357:851–62.

[4] Grossman I, Nili A, Singer C, et al. Pharmacogenetics of glatiramer acetate therapy for multiple sclerosis reveals drug-response markers. Pharmacogenet Genomics 2007;17:657–66.

[5] Taylor TN, Davis PH, Torner JC, et al. Lifetime cost of stroke in the United States. Stroke 1996;27:1459–66.

[6] Matarin M, Brown MM, Scholz S, et al. A genome-wide genotyping study in patients with ischaemic stroke: initial analysis and data release. Lancet Neurol 2007;6:414–20.

[7] Lalouschek W, Endler G, Schillinger M, et al. Candidate genetic risk factors of stroke: results of a multilocus genotyping assay. Clin Chem 2007;53:600–5.

[8] Jerrard-Dunne P, Markus HS, Steckel DA, et al. Early carotid atherosclerosis and family history of vascular disease: specific effects on arterial sites have implications for genetic studies. Arterioscler Thromb Vasc Biol 2003;23:302–6.

[9] Humphries SE, Morgan L. Genetic risk factors for stroke and carotid atherosclerosis: insights into pathophysiology from candidate gene approaches [review] [134 refs]. Lancet Neurol 2004;3:227–35.

[10] Greisenegger S, Endler G, Haering D, et al. The (-174) G/C polymorphism in the interleukin-6 gene

is associated with the severity of acute cerebrovascular events. Thromb Res 2003;110:181–6.

[11] Lee BC, Ahn SY, Doo HK, et al. Susceptibility for ischemic stroke in Korean population is associated with polymorphisms of the interleukin-1 receptor antagonist and tumor necrosis factor-alpha genes, but not the interleukin-1beta gene. Neurosci Lett 2004;357:33.

[12] Worrall BB, Brott TG, Brown RD Jr, et al. IL1RN VNTR polymorphism in ischemic stroke: analysis in 3 populations. Stroke 2007;38:1189–96.

[13] Pola R, Flex A, Gaetani E, et al. Synergistic effect of -174 G/C polymorphism of the interleukin-6 gene promoter and 469 E/K polymorphism of the intercellular adhesion molecule-1 gene in Italian patients with history of ischemic stroke. Stroke 2003;34:881–5.

[14] Um JY, An NH, Kim HM. TNF-alpha and TNF-beta gene polymorphisms in cerebral infarction. J Mol Neurosci 2003;21:167–71.

[15] Um JY, Moon KS, Lee KM, et al. Interleukin-1 gene cluster polymorphisms in cerebral infarction. Cytokine 2003;23:41–6.

[16] Um JY, Moon KS, Lee KM, et al. Association of interleukin-1 alpha gene polymorphism with cerebral infarction. Brain Res Mol Brain Res 2003;115:50–4.

[17] Zee RY, Cook NR, Cheng S, et al. Polymorphism in the P-selectin and interleukin-4 genes as determinants of stroke: a population-based, prospective genetic analysis. Hum Mol Genet 2004;13:389–96.

[18] Morita A, Nakayama T, Soma M. Association study between C-reactive protein genes and ischemic stroke in Japanese subjects. Am J Hypertens 2006;19:593–600.

[19] Colaizzo DA, Fofi LB, Tiscia GA, et al. The COX-2 G/C -765 polymorphism may modulate the occurrence of cerebrovascular ischemia [article]. Blood Coagul Fibrinolysis 2006;17:93–6.

[20] Cronin S, Furie KL, Kelly PJ. Dose-related association of MTHFR 677T allele with risk of ischemic stroke: evidence from a cumulative meta-analysis [see comment]. Stroke 2005;36:1581–7.

[21] Gretarsdottir S, Sveinbjornsdottir S, Jonsson HH, et al. Localization of a susceptibility gene for common forms of stroke to 5q12. Am J Hum Genet 2002;70:593–603.

[22] Gretarsdottir S, Thorleifsson G, Reynisdottir ST, et al. The gene encoding phosphodiesterase 4D confers risk of ischemic stroke [see comment] [erratum appears in Nat Genet. 2005 May;37(5):555]. Nat Genet 2003;35:131–8.

[23] Fidani L, Clarimon J, Goulas A, et al. Association of phosphodiesterase 4D gene G0 haplotype and ischaemic stroke in a Greek population. Eur J Neurol 2007;14:745–9.

[24] Meschia JF, Brott TG, Brown RD Jr, et al. Phosphodiesterase 4D and 5-lipoxygenase activating protein in ischemic stroke. Ann Neurol 2005;58:351–61.

[25] Nakayama T, Asai S, Sato N, et al. Genotype and haplotype association study of the STRK1 region on 5q12 among Japanese: a case-control study. Stroke 2006;37:69–76.

[26] Sun L, Li Z, Zhang H, et al. Pentanucleotide TTTTA repeat polymorphism of apolipoprotein(a) gene and plasma lipoprotein(a) are associated with ischemic and hemorrhagic stroke in Chinese: a multicenter case-control study in China. Stroke 2003;34:1617–22.

[27] Szolnoki Z, Havasi V, Talian G, et al. Lymphotoxin-alpha gene 252G allelic variant is a risk factor for large-vessel-associated ischemic stroke. J Mol Neurosci 2005;27:205–11.

[28] Shimo-Nakanishi Y, Urabe T, Hattori N, et al. Polymorphism of the lipoprotein lipase gene and risk of atherothrombotic cerebral infarction in the Japanese. Stroke 2001;32:1481–6.

[29] Rubattu S, Di Angelantonio E, Stanzione R, et al. Gene polymorphisms of the renin-angiotensin-aldosterone system and the risk of ischemic stroke: a role of the A1166C/AT1 gene variant. J Hypertens 2004;22:2129–34.

[30] Cole JW, Roberts SC, Gallagher M, et al. Thrombomodulin Ala455Val polymorphism and the risk of cerebral infarction in a biracial population: the Stroke Prevention in Young Women Study. BMC Neurol 2004;4:1–21.

[31] Szolnoki Z, Somogyvari F, Kondacs A, et al. Increased prevalence of platelet glycoprotein IIb/IIIa PLA2 allele in ischaemic stroke associated with large vessel pathology. Thromb Res 2003;109:265–9.

[32] Jood K, Ladenvall P, Tjarnlund-Wolf A, et al. Fibrinolytic gene polymorphism and ischemic stroke. Stroke 2005;36:2077–81.

[33] Voetsch B, Jin RC, Bierl C, et al. Promoter polymorphisms in the plasma glutathione peroxidase (GPx-3) gene: a novel risk factor for arterial ischemic stroke among young adults and children [see comment]. Stroke 2007;38:41–9.

[34] Howard TD, Giles WH, Xu J, et al. Promoter polymorphisms in the nitric oxide synthase 3 gene are associated with ischemic stroke susceptibility in young black women. Stroke 2005;36:1848–51.

[35] Szolnoki Z, Havasi V, Bene J, et al. Endothelial nitric oxide synthase gene interactions and the risk of ischaemic stroke. Acta Neurol Scand 2005;111:29–33.

[36] Rubattu S, Stanzione R, Di Angelantonio E, et al. Atrial natriuretic peptide gene polymorphisms and risk of ischemic stroke in humans. Stroke 2004;35:814–8.

[37] Casas JP, Hingorani AD, Bautista LE, et al. Meta-analysis of genetic studies in ischemic stroke: thirty-two genes involving approximately 18,000 cases and 58,000 controls. Arch Neurol 2004;61:1652–61.

[38] Lalouschek W, Schillinger M, Hsieh K, et al. Matched case-control study on factor V Leiden and the prothrombin G20210A mutation in patients with ischemic stroke/transient ischemic attack up to the age of 60 years. Stroke 2005;36:1405–9.

[39] Li C, Zhang C, Qiu S, et al. Polymorphisms of ACE-1 and MTHFR genes and genetic susceptibility of ischemic stroke. Zhonghua Yi Xue Za Zhi 2002;82:1046–9.

[40] Morita H, Kurihara H, Tsubaki S, et al. Methylene-tetrahydrofolate reductase gene polymorphism and ischemic stroke in Japanese. Arterioscler Thromb Vasc Biol 1998;18:1465–9.

[41] McCarron MO, Delong D, Alberts MJ. APOE genotype as a risk factor for ischemic cerebrovascular disease: a meta-analysis. Neurology 1999;53:1308–11.

[42] Margaglione M, Seripa D, Gravina C, et al. Prevalence of apolipoprotein E alleles in healthy subjects and survivors of ischemic stroke: an Italian case-control study. Stroke 1998;29:399–403.

[43] Peng DQ, Zhao SP, Wang JL. Lipoprotein (a) and apolipoprotein E epsilon 4 as independent risk factors for ischemic stroke. J Cardiovasc Risk 1999;6:1–6.

[44] Barr TL, Conley YP. Poly(ADP-ribose) polymerase-1 and its clinical applications in brain injury. J Neurosci Nurs 2007;39:278–84.

[45] Takahashi K, Pieper AA, Croul SE, et al. Post treatment with an inhibitor of poly(ADP-ribose)polymerase attenuates cerebral damage in focal ischemia. Brain Res 1999;829:46–54.

[46] Gemmati D, Serino ML, Ongaro A, et al. A common mutation in the gene for coagulation factor XIII-A (VAL34Leu): a risk factor for primary intracerebral hemorrhage is protective against athero-thrombotic diseases. Am J Hematol 2001;67:183–8.

[47] Kokubo Y, Chowdhury AH, Date C, et al. Age-dependent association of apolipoprotein E genotypes with stroke subtypes in a Japanese rural population. Stroke 2000;31:1299–306.

[48] Peters DG, Kassam A, St Jean PL, et al. Functional polymorphism in the matrix metalloproteinase-9 promoter as a potential risk factor for intracranial aneurysm. Stroke 1999;30:2612–9.

[49] Khurana VG, Sohni YR, Mangrum WI, et al. Endothelial nitric oxide synthase gene polymorphisms predict susceptibility to aneurysmal subarachnoid hemorrhage and cerebral vasospasm. J Cereb Blood Flow Metab 2004;24:291–7.

[50] Fisher C, Kistler J, Davis J. Relation of cerebral vasospasm to subarachnoid hemorrhage visualized by computerized tomographic scanning. Neurosurgery 1980;6(1):1–9.

[51] Vergouwen MD, Frijns CJ, Roos YB, et al. Plasminogen inhibitor-1 4G allele in the 4G/5G promoter polymorphism increases the occurrence of cerebral ischemia after aneurysmal subarachnoid hemorrhage. Stroke 2004;35:1280–3.

[52] Ruigrok YM, Slooter AJ, Bardoel A, et al. Genes and outcome after aneurysmal subarachnoid haemorrhage. J Neurol 2005;252:417–22.

[53] Muller W, Meske V, Berlin K, et al. Apolipoprotein E isoforms increase intracellular Ca2+ differentially through a omega-agatoxin IVa-sensitive Ca2+-channel. Brain Pathol 1998;8:641–53.

[54] Tolar M, Keller JN, Chan S, et al. Truncated apolipoprotein E (ApoE) causes increased intracellular calcium and may mediate ApoE neurotoxicity. J Neurosci 1999;19:7100–10.

[55] Veinbergs I, Everson A, Sagara Y, et al. Neurotoxic effects of apolipoprotein E4 are mediated via dysregulation of calcium homeostasis. J Neurosci Res 2002;67:379–87.

[56] Hayashi H, Igbavboa U, Hamanaka H, et al. Cholesterol is increased in the exofacial leaflet of synaptic plasma membranes of human apolipoprotein E4 knock-in mice. Neuroreport 2002;13:383–6.

[57] Mauch DH, Nagler K, Schumacher S, et al. CNS synaptogenesis promoted by glia-derived cholesterol. Science 2001;294:1354–7.

[58] Nathan BP, Bellosta S, Sanan DA, et al. Differential effects of apolipoproteins E3 and E4 on neuronal growth in vitro. Science 1994;264:850–2.

[59] Mahley RW. Apolipoprotein E: cholesterol transport protein with expanding role in cell biology [review] [99 refs]. Science 1988;240:622–30.

[60] Weisgraber KH. Apolipoprotein E: structure-function relationships [review] [201 refs]. Adv Protein Chem 1994;45:249–302.

[61] Lanterna LA, Ruigrok Y, Alexander S, et al. Meta-analysis of APOE genotype and subarachnoid hemorrhage: clinical outcome and delayed ischemia. Neurology 2007;69:766–75.

[62] Liaquat I, Dunn LT, Nicoll JA, et al. Effect of apolipoprotein E genotype on hematoma volume after trauma. J Neurosurg 2002;96:90–6.

[63] Lynch JR, Pineda JA, Morgan D, et al. Apolipoprotein E affects the central nervous system response to injury and the development of cerebral edema. Ann Neurol 2002;51:113–7.

[64] Nicoll JA, Roberts GW, Graham DI. Amyloid beta-protein, APOE genotype and head injury [review] [9 refs]. Ann N Y Acad Sci 1996;777:271–5.

[65] Teasdale GM, Nicoll JA, Murray G, et al. Association of apolipoprotein E polymorphism with outcome after head injury. Lancet 1997;350:1069–71.

[66] Kerr ME, Ilyas Kamboh M, Yookyung K, et al. Relationship between apoE4 allele and excitatory amino acid levels after traumatic brain injury. Crit Care Med 2003;31:2371–9.

[67] Kerr ME, Kamboh MI, Kong Y, et al. Apolipoprotein E genotype and CBF in traumatic brain injured patients. Adv Exp Med Biol 2006;578:291–6.

[68] Csuka E, Morganti-Kossmann MC, Lenzlinger PM, et al. IL-10 levels in cerebrospinal fluid and serum of patients with severe traumatic brain injury: relationship to IL-6, TNF-alpha, TGF-beta1 and blood-brain barrier function. J Neuroimmunol 1999;101:211–21.

[69] Wichterle J, Lieberam I, Porter JA, et al. Directed differentiation of embryonic stem cells into motor neurons. Cell 2002;110:385–97.

[70] Cao QL, Benton RL, Whittemore SR. Stem cell repair of central nervous system injury. J Neurosci Res 2002;68:501–10.

[71] Cao QL, Howard RM, Dennison JB, et al. Differentiation of engrafted neuronal-restricted precursor cells is inhibited in the traumatically injured spinal cord. Exp Neurol 2002;177:349–59.

ELSEVIER
SAUNDERS

Crit Care Nurs Clin N Am 20 (2008) 213–221

CRITICAL CARE
NURSING CLINICS
OF NORTH AMERICA

Inflammation and Genomics in the Critical Care Unit

Chris Winkelman, RN, PhD, CCRN, ACNP

*Frances Payne Bolton School of Nursing, Case Western Reserve University, 10900 Euclid Avenue,
Cleveland, OH 44206, USA*

Inflammation is a physiologic response to irritants, injury, and infection. In early historical medical records, inflammation is characterized by redness, swelling, heat, and pain; in the 19th century Virchow added loss of function as a fifth defining component [1]. As a fundamental biologic response of cells and tissue to harmful stimuli, inflammation contributes to the dilution, destruction, or containment of pathogens and injured tissue [2]. Once initiated, the inflammatory syndrome proceeds in a complex biologic cascade that is typically short lived and self-limited. At times, however, inflammatory processes proceed from appropriate localized reactions to inappropriate systemic responses or persist beyond the usual hours or days needed for a healthy immunologic response. Systemic and persistent inflammation is believed to contribute to morbidity and mortality from many diseases and is the focus of genomic research in critical illness.

This article reviews the approaches used to investigate the molecular biology of inflammation, providing insight into the onset, normal progression, and pathogenesis. Findings from molecular investigations have significant potential to contribute to diagnostic and clinical treatment of pathology that has challenged critical care providers for decades, including severe trauma, massive burns, and sepsis. Although this information does not yet translate into direct care applications, clinicians, researchers, and educators will benefit from increasing their familiarity with genomic terminology and appreciating the bench-to-bedside progress in understanding complex patient responses to irritants, injury, and infection. Early identification of dysfunctional inflammation

using genomically derived biomarkers has the potential to promote new interventions and better outcomes among critically ill patients.

Molecular genetic approaches to investigate inflammation

There is wide variation in individual response to irritants, injury, and infection. For example, some individuals are hyperresponsive, mounting an impressive inflammatory reaction to a minor viral infection or skin irritant. Premature death from infections has been genetically linked to high levels of serum proinflammatory factors [3]. Host response has been investigated with various genomic techniques, including use of phenotypic-genetic linkage (linkage analysis), determinations of expression patterns from mRNA (transcriptome analysis), and exploration of patterns of released proteins and protein activity (proteome analysis). New statistical and pathway models have been developed to manage the large volume of data from these experiments and to compare data between experiments. To understand the results of investigations that focus on inflammation, an explanation of the various molecular approaches with associated strengths and limitations is first described.

When first attempting to identify a specific gene or genes responsible for a problem, the investigator selects a region of a chromosome that has been linked or associated with the problem under investigation. Genes in a selected chromosomal region that are also biologically plausible are termed "candidate genes." Many candidate genes are located from known single-gene or mendelian conditions, whereas others are located because the protein products produced by that region have been studied extensively. For

E-mail address: chris.winkelman@case.edu

example, we know where the gene for producing insulin and other products used in glucose metabolism are located. In trying to determine the different inherited factors leading to the development of type II diabetes, it would be logical to examine the genes responsible for glucose metabolism and use, such as the insulin gene, the insulin receptor gene, the gene (or genes) for membrane glucose transport proteins, and those genes for the enzymes involved in the glycolytic pathway and the Krebs cycle. Many of the candidate genes for inflammation are along chromosome 6, which carries the code for many immunologic proteins.

Linkage analysis

Linkage analysis is used to identify the location of a gene that is associated with disease or other variation of the human condition. A modification of this approach allows researchers to locate any associated alleles, which are minor variations in genes. With linkage analysis, genetic researchers locate markers of disease (or inflammatory dysfunction) by examining the relationship between two factors, such as two known traits, two known genetic markers, or a known trait and a known genetic marker. For example, common human traits that are typically inherited together are male gender and ear hair. Genetic linkage analysis established that the gene coding for ear hair is located on chromosome Y, the same chromosome that determines male gender. Women thus do not grow ear hair. Although this is a light-hearted example of linkage analysis, investigations into inflammation have used this type of linkage analysis to locate variations in DNA sequences that link inflammatory function to normal and aberrant inflammatory responses.

Variations in the DNA sequence are polymorphisms. One type of genomic variation is the single nucleotide polymorphism (SNP)—a single base pair substitution in the gene sequence of DNA. Another common polymorphism is a variation in the length of a repetitive DNA sequence in a coding region. Variable repeats are labeled microsatellites or variable number of tandem repeats depending on the location and number of repetitive sequences. Polymorphisms can affect gene transcription, RNA stability, and the activity of the resultant protein [4]. Although not all polymorphisms result in differences among individuals, the extent of an individual inflammatory response can vary depending on the presence of SNPs or repeated sequences of DNA. Further,

the inheritance of a single gene or two gene alleles with important variations—homozygous or heterozygous alleles—contributes to individual inflammatory responsiveness.

Most genetic association studies examine candidate genes with single polymorphisms. As a result of the Human Genome Project, the technology to detect SNPs has become increasingly standardized and accessible, leading to an explosion of reports investigating how inherited factors influence the onset and progression of many health problems, including the syndrome of inflammation and its related processes. Initially, technology for genetic linkage analysis allowed investigation of only a few SNPs at one time; genotyping chips that allow simultaneous identification of 500 to 50,000 SNPs are in trial now. With single-gene diseases, variations in a single coding region of a gene on one chromosome result in pathology; isolating a few SNPs was a reasonable, cost-effective method to identify genetic contributions. In a cascade as complex as inflammation, the contributions of SNPs within one coding region are more challenging to identify and interpret. Two regions have produced intriguing results: (1) genes that control the production of small molecules, such as cytokines, in the inflammatory cascade, and (2) the coding DNA that precedes these genes—the area preceding a gene known as the promoter region, which "turns on" the gene and initiates production of the gene product. To illustrate, tumor necrosis factor-alpha (TNF-α) is an important molecular factor in the inflammatory cascade. High levels of serum TNF-α are associated with an increased occurrence of shock and death in septic patients [5,6]. TNF-α polymorphisms have also been associated with increased risk for inflammatory dysregulation in burn and trauma patients [7,8]. Along with polymorphisms in the gene that codes for TNF-α, polymorphisms within the promoter region for the TNF-α gene are believed to contribute to progression to septic shock in systemic infection among critically ill adults [9].

Genes coding for other proinflammatory and anti-inflammatory factors have been investigated for contributions to the intensity or moderation of the inflammatory response. Other genes that code for proteins are used to recognize pathogens or to alter intravascular dynamics and add to our understanding of host response to irritants, injury, and infection. These candidate genes and their protein products are summarized in Table 1. Although many of the findings from investigations

Table 1
Selected genes and their products implicated in variant human inflammatory response

Gene	Molecule/factor	Role in inflammation
TNFA OMIM 191160	Tumor necrosis factor	Proinflammatory
IL1B OMIM 147720	Interleukin-1β	Proinflammatory
IL1RN OMIM 147810	Interleukin-1 receptor antagonist	Anti-inflammatory
IL6 OMIM 147620	Interleukin-6	Proinflammatory with concurrent anti-inflammatory properties
IL10 OMIM 124092	Interleukin-10	Anti-inflammatory
PAI1 OMIM 173360	Plasma activator inhibitor type 1	Antifibrinolytic proinflammatory
HSF1 OMIM 140580	Heat shock protein transcription factor	Proinflammatory
TLR4 OMIM 603030	Toll-like receptor 4	Proinflammatory
F5 OMIM 227400	Factor V Leiden	Coagulant proinflammatory
IFNG OMIM 147570	Interferon-gamma	Proinflammatory

Data from Winning et al. Molecular biology in the ICU. Minerva Anesthesiol 2006;72:255–67; and NCBI. Online Mendelian inheritance in man. August 27, 2007. Available at: http://www.ncbi.nlm.nih.gov/sites/entrez. Accessed September 1, 2007.

of human inflammation that use linkage analysis are underpowered, they provide important genomic information about the inheritable multiplicity of host responses to irritants, infection, and injury [10].

Linkage analysis has several limitations, especially in polygenic, multifactorial syndromes like inflammation. Subtleties in the phenotype, genetic and environmental modifiers, and hidden features, such a variable penetrance or mosaicism, may make it difficult to locate important contributions from a single gene. Inflammatory response is not only the result of multiple variations within a coding region; it is also polygenic. Multiple genes across several chromosomes contribute to the inflammatory cascade. Methods that simultaneously investigate multiple polymorphisms have the potential to better describe complex genomics. Functional investigations using transcriptome and proteome approaches that include a clinical context will help genomic researchers detail inflammatory processes.

Transcriptome analysis

Another approach to describe inflammatory responses is to examine the differences in populations of mRNA between health and disease [11]. Conversely, other expression patterns may be associated with better responses to treatment regimens. Transcriptome analysis uses microarrays and quantitative fluorescent labeling to screen for changes in the amount of mRNA associated with thousands of genes after a single event in one subject. Multiple microarrays from different samples are then compared with each other. Genes with high expression of mRNA are identified with statistical methods. These data are then used to profile the genes and the pathways activated by the stimulus. This technology is already being used in some cancer settings to classify breast tumors; specific expression patterns of mRNA expressed by biopsied tumor tissue can be associated with poor prognosis [12]. In critically ill patients, transcriptome analysis is being used to identify clusters of coexpressed genes that regulate inflammation by identifying mRNA.

One goal with transcriptome analysis is to determine whether gene expression score can reliably predict aberrant inflammation. Initial steps are to identify similarities and differences between systemic inflammatory patterns of expression in common pathologies, such as trauma, burns, and sepsis. Generally, a case control design is used; patient samples are matched for time postadmission, time to systemic inflammation, and demographic and clinical data (such as steroid use/dose); then the differences between subjects with normal responses and abnormal systemic inflammation are examined.

One concern with microarray transcriptome analysis is that changes in the volume of mRNA do not necessarily correlate with changes in the amount of protein synthesized. Adding to the challenge of interpreting findings of microarrays, the variations within an individual in response to injury or infection are wide, making comparisons across subjects challenging. At this time, a whole-genome approach to transcriptome analysis is not available; examining only a few selected mRNAs may skew pathway analyses. Severity of dysfunctional inflammation and differences between early and late dysfunction are not well characterized and may confound the interpretation of findings from microarray technology [11,13]. Transcriptome analysis holds promise in identifying functions of proteins but protein quantity and type need to be better understood to fulfill that promise. Another approach to elucidate conditions of health and disease during inflammation is proteome analysis.

Proteome analysis

A third approach to investigating the human response of inflammation is to quantify the various proteins produced after inflammatory stimuli. Cellular proteins vary tremendously in volume, especially in body fluids. For example, albumin is measured in milligrams per milliliter, whereas TNF-α is measured in picograms per milliliter—a difference of 10^{-9}. Finding one platform that can determine differences in the volume of multiple proteins with a single analysis is challenging. Nonetheless, analytic techniques in liquid chromatography, mass spectrometry, and two-dimensional electrophoresis do provide data for hundreds to thousands of proteins simultaneously [14].

More typically, proteome analysis for inflammation uses immunoassays that can detect low volumes of a specific protein in tissue or body fluid. This technique uses a specific antibody to detect and measure a molecular factor. After enzymatically binding to the inflammatory molecular protein, the antibody–antigen complex generates a signal, often fluorescent, that can be measured. In general, the immunoassays that examine inflammatory molecules are noncompetitive (sandwich) methods that use two highly specific antibody reagents to bind to the protein of interest, essentially sandwiching the protein between the two antibodies. These assays can only measure one protein at a time and provide limited information about the function of that protein within the cell or tissue [15].

Findings from linkage analyses in inflammation and critical illnesses

Genetic variants in important inflammatory mediators have been described in more than 100 reports of linkage analysis in human subjects. Findings include polymorphisms that code for pathogen detection receptors, cytokines, inflammatory receptors, intracellular signaling cascades, heat shock proteins, coagulation/fibrinolysis pathways, apoptotic mechanisms, and neuroendocrine function. Unfortunately, findings have been inconsistent, with insufficient numbers of subjects to determine the levels needed to rule out false-positive results [10]. Combined with methodologic and analytic problems that result in the inability to replicate results, conclusive evidence for specific genetic contributions to inflammatory dysfunction has yet to be determined. Nonetheless, mediators and candidate genes identified through linkage analysis suggest that genetic factors play an important role in the pathology of persistent or prolonged inflammation in critically ill adults.

Findings from transcriptome analyses

Transcriptome analysis is a newer genomic methodology and has fewer supporting data for detailing human inflammatory responses compared with linkage analysis. Three studies illustrate the value of this approach to profiling inflammatory responses. McDunn and colleagues [11] report the results of microarray analyses from five subjects who had abdominal pain. Their hypothesis, based on animal data, was that differences in circulating leukocyte mRNA would distinguish inflammatory/infectious sources of abdominal pain from noninfectious sources. Subjects who had no-to-intermediate levels of cytokines did not require surgery; the two subjects who had elevated ratios of interleukin (IL)–6 to IL-7 or IL-12 to granulocyte-macrophage colony-stimulating factor required surgical intervention. The authors suggest that further validation of the findings from microarray analyses could provide new diagnostic tools for the clinician, especially in the presence of ambiguous or uncertain data from conventional assessments [11].

Chung and colleagues [16] report on 12 subjects who had sepsis, proposing that splenic genes would be differentially expressed in the presence of sterile (ie, trauma- or surgery-induced) versus infectious (ie, bacterial- or fungal-induced) systemic inflammation. "Considerable" differences between septic and injured patients were demonstrated in microarray analysis; however, there was also considerable variation within septic and injured patients. With the large interindividual variation and the small sample size, no individual genes were identified as specifically contributing to one profile of inflammation. The authors were able to build a predictive model of sterile versus infectious inflammation from microarray results that robustly predicted inflammatory profiles in mice. Importantly, it was the pattern of changes in gene expression, not the magnitude of change, that provided predictive data. Information about patterned change could help the clinician quickly identify patients in the ICU who need closer monitoring or who are not responding to conventional interventions.

Using transcriptome methodology, these researchers analyzed serum from 50 subjects who had inflammation in four different intensive care units. Results included differential expression of 131 unique gene activities in patients who had documented sepsis compared with bypass surgery patients who did not have clinical indicators for sepsis. A total of 1236 additional genes were similarly expressed in all patients; these might be considered the "normal" genetic expression after an inflammatory event such as surgery and sepsis [17].

Two large studies are currently in progress using microarray technology to observe the genomic expression of inflammatory proteins after severe injury and infection. Inflammation and the Host Response to Injury, sponsored by the National Institute of General Medical Sciences, focuses on injured and burn patients and the development of sepsis (http://www.gluegrant.org). In Germany, a related large study is looking at leukocyte response and genomic expression in patients who are at high risk for sepsis (German National Genome Research Network; http://www.ngfn.de/ngfn_en/index.html). Federal funding for studies examining inflammation in humans with microarray technology includes investigation of acute lung injury, cardiovascular tissue, and liver tissue after transplant (http://crisp.cit.nih.gov/crisp/CRISP; search terms microarray and inflammation).

Findings from proteomics

The exponential growth in identifying mediators of inflammation is related to the refinement of laboratory techniques that allow detection of extremely small quantities of intra- and intercellular proteins. Along with identifying small inflammatory proteins, advances in bench analyses have contributed to our understanding of protein activity, including compartmentalization, complexation, posttranslational modification, and degradation. The newest techniques promise to further classify proteins as membrane, nuclear,

and ribosomal; such data can be used in diagnostics and targeted therapy. More than 500,000 proteins are believed to be synthesized by human genes; posttranslational modifications are hypothesized to bring the total number of human proteins to more than 2 million (US Human Proteome Organization; http://www.ushupo.org). Because proteins are essential to life, understanding the structure and function of proteins will clarify complex pathways and develop a deep understanding of the inflammatory cascade.

There are several families of proteins that serve as biomarkers for inflammation. These families have several interconnected mechanisms that initiate and sustain inflammation. These families include vasoactive amines, complement, defensins, procoagulation factors, fibrinolytic factors and kinins, prostaglandins, leukotrienes, and cytokines. Some of these soluble proteins are present at a constant rate regardless of physiologic demand or the concentration of a substrate (ie, constitutively expressed) in plasma or other biologic fluids. Other biomarkers of inflammation are synthesized and released from cells in response to a stimulus. For most of these proteins, when they are present in the plasma either constitutively or only in response to a stimulus, they are inactive until triggered. Inflammatory proteins may thus exist in plasma without causing inflammation, instead acting as growth factors or promoting other functions. Once triggered or activated, inflammatory proteins interact with various cells, promoting the inflammatory cascade directly and stimulating production of additional inflammatory proteins. Generally, leukocytes are the primary source of inflammatory proteins, although all nucleated cells possess the genes that code for inflammatory protein synthesis. These soluble proteins and their function in inflammation are summarized below.

Vasoactive amines

The vasoactive amines are fast-acting mediators that influence the immediate response to irritation, invasion, or injury. Many amines are synthesized in specialized leukocytes and stored in granules until a stimulus for release occurs. One example is a product of mast cells and basophils: histamine. When intracellular granules of histamine are released, local blood vessels dilate and capillaries become more permeable, leading to warmth, redness, and swelling at the site of inflammation. Variations in the amount and location of amine release lead to the variable inflammatory response in skin, airways, and mucous membranes [18–20].

Complement

The complement proteins are small bioactive molecules manufactured primarily by the liver. Monocytes also contribute to the synthesis of circulating complement proteins. Complement includes 30 plasma and cell-surface proteins and is associated with both up-regulating and down-regulating inflammation pathways. Complement proteins act to opsonize or coat microbes for recognition and removal by monocytes and macrophages. They also recruit phagocytes and contribute to lytic destruction of pathogens. Even small fragments of some complement factors promote inflammatory responses by stimulating bone marrow release of granulocytes and acting as a chemoattractant for monocytes, neutrophils, and eosinophils at localized infections. Activated complement proteins stimulate release of histamine along with indirectly contributing to the synthesis and release of cytokines, further contributing to inflammatory symptoms [21–23].

Defensins

Defensins are small peptides synthesized in neutrophils, epithelial cells of the mucous membranes and intestines, and in skin cells. They are antimicrobial, stimulating disruption of the microbial pathogen cell walls. These small proteins also promote inflammation by posttranslation processing of IL-1β and as chemoattractants for neutrophils, mast cells, memory T cells, and immature dendritic cells. In addition, β-defensins may contribute to the activation and maturation of dendritic cells [24].

Coagulants and fibrinolytics

The interactions between the inflammatory and the coagulation cascades result in a procoagulative status and a disruption of the fibrinolytic response that leads to microcirculation impairment. Among critically ill adults, there is a link between activated protein C and reduced mortality from sepsis, but the mechanism by which this anticoagulant works to promote a good outcome is not clear [25]. Further investigation, using genomic technology, is helping to elucidate the interactions between inflammation and coagulation.

One component of the coagulation cascade implicated as a mediator of inflammation is plasminogen activator inhibitor type-1(PAI-1). It has a dual role of acting as an acute phase protein in periods of acute inflammation and in inhibiting, as it name implies, the conversion of plasminogen into its active form, stopping the clotting process. High levels of PAI-1 contribute to disseminated intravascular coagulopathy by shutting down the fibrinolytic system so that microvascular fibrin clots cannot be dissolved. High levels of circulating PAI-1 are associated with poor outcomes, increased severity of disease, and increased levels of proinflammatory cytokines and acute phase proteins in patients who have sepsis [26].

Prostaglandins

Prostaglandins are found in nearly every human tissue. They are the result of enzymatic transformation of arachidonic acid released from the lipid layers of cell membranes. There are prostaglandin receptors on various tissues and some of these ligand-activated receptors contribute to inflammation. Selected prostaglandins also cause vasodilation or vasoconstriction, smooth muscle constriction, platelet aggregation, sensitization of neurons to pain, calcium movement into cells, and hormone regulation, and influence growth factors for cell repair [27,28].

Leukotrienes

When cell membranes release arachidonic acid, an endogenous enzyme, lipoxygenase, converts this substance to leukotrienes. Leukotrienes act to sustain inflammation. For example, one subfamily of leukotrienes (ie, LTB4) is a chemoattractant, serving to bring migrating neutrophils to the site of inflammation. Leukocytes have receptors for the subfamilies of leukotrienes; when leukotrienes are attached to these receptors the white cells are activated, synthesizing additional inflammatory factors and other factors involved in host defense. Other leukotrienes bind to tissue and smooth muscle, causing vasoconstriction and bronchoconstriction, which serve to contain injury or irritants [29].

Cytokines and chemokines

Cytokines are small proteins that derive their name from their potent role in the inflammatory response: cell-to-cell communication. They are components of a complex network that is involved in almost every pathway related to inflammation. Cytokines include ILs, interferons, growth factors, and chemokines. Several excellent reviews of cytokines have been published [30–34]. Currently, 70 different cytokines have been proposed [33]. The type and amounts of cytokines produced vary in response to time of day, duration of stimulus, variations in the cellular environment of the synthesizing cells, and other factors. Which cytokines are produced in response to an irritant, injury, or infectious agent influences innate and cell-mediated immune responses. Further, a cytokine may be pluripotent, differing in function depending on its source, target, and the phase of the immune response in which it is released [31]. For example, IL-6 is both proinflammatory and anti-inflammatory. It induces fever and the synthesis of acute phase proteins in the liver—clearly properties promoting and sustaining inflammation. IL-6 also inhibits inflammation, however, by reducing upstream synthesis of TNF and IL-1; reduced levels of TNF and IL-1 result in down-regulation of inflammation. Cytokines of particular interest to critical care researchers and practitioners include TNF, IL-1, IL-6, and the anti-inflammatory, IL-10. These interleukins have been found to have important associations with the severity and progression of trauma syndromes, such as acute lung injury and multiorgan dysfunction, cardiovascular disease, and sepsis [35–38]. Other cytokines have been associated with specific disease processes that are often found in critically ill patients, such as macrophage migration inhibitory factor (MIF). MIF is constitutively synthesized by various cells and tissues; production and release of this inflammatory mediator is rapidly increased after exposure to microbial cell wall components and toxins. MIF is implicated in the pathogenesis of sepsis, acute lung injury, and acute renal failure [39]. Further investigation is needed to clearly understand how the internal milieu of the host with an immune insult affects the function and interaction of these potent inflammatory molecules [40].

Toll-like receptors

Along with these soluble proteins, there are membrane-bound proteins that influence the host response to inflammatory stimuli. Toll-like receptors (TLRs) are major sensors of bacteria in humans and other mammals, insects, and plants. TLRs are important in stimulating inflammatory cytokine responses, including IL-12 and IL-23 secretions. Ten different types of TLRs are defined in humans. Altered or lack of TLR may play a role in the regulatory responses of humans to infection [23,41].

Genetic inheritance is not the sole determinant of an individual's inflammatory response. One's internal environment, influenced by diet, age, gender, endocrine function, and central nervous system signals also promote and sustain inflammation. External environmental factors, such as time of day, virulence of an invading microorganism, and the size of the inoculums, also influence inflammatory pathways and molecules. Environmental factors may be protective; childhood exposure to helminths is associated with down-regulation of inflammation and may prevent pathologic immune reactivity leading to inflammatory bowel disease in later years [42]. Other environmental stimuli may be harmful, contributing to autoimmune disease. Inflammatory dysregulation is just one example in complex genomic investigation. Sorting the contributions of genetics and environment may not be possible. Genomic technology has advanced our knowledge of the structure and function of inflammatory molecules, however, and helped to provide insight into the pathways that result in physiologic, protective inflammation and aberrant inflammatory responses as with allergies or idiopathic immunosuppression. Animal models, especially knockout mice, continue to provide new data about inflammation.

Additional approaches investigating inflammation in critical illnesses

Knockout mice are one more genomic "technology" used to develop knowledge about host inflammatory responses. A knockout mouse is a laboratory mouse that has an inactivated (knocked out) gene. Stopping the activity of a gene provides information about what the gene does and how the absence of a gene contributes to disease (http://www.genome.gov/12514551). More information about how knockout mice are produced can be found at the Web site of the Human Genome Project. Mice that do not have the gene to produce TNF-α have been studied extensively. Without TNF-α, mice are less likely to have inflammatory responses to transplanted organs and to irritants like asbestos. These mice do not develop an immune response to TB or abnormal (ie, cancer) cells, however [43].

Another emerging approach to genomics is computational biology—new statistical models to identify and predict the contributions of genes to complex conditions of health and disease. Because generational documentation does not have the same informative value as with single-gene or mendelian traits, determining the model for the volume and complexity of data generated by transcriptome and proteome analyses has led to new and specialized statistics. Describing these new models is beyond the scope of this article but several primers are available to the novice, including one developed by scientists for the Human Genome Project (http://www.ncbi.nlm.nih.gov/About/primer/molecularmod.html) [44].

Implications for nurses

Knowledge of genetic factors that influence human inflammatory syndromes is providing new insight into both normal and abnormal responses to irritants, injury, and infection. The results of these investigations may lead to treatments to modify aberrant inflammation while allowing normal inflammatory regulation to protect uninjured and uninfected cells, tissues, and organs, assisting repair and recovery. Nurses should include previous history or responses to infections and injury to better understand individual inflammatory syndromes.

Findings from genomic studies better characterize the interplay between patient characteristics, such as age or gender, and environmental factors, such as time of day or diet, that influence inflammatory response. Nurses who are aware of genomic findings that quantify these influential factors may be more alert to early symptoms and provide information to alter modifiable risk factors. Determining patterns of abnormal responses or biomarkers early in the course of a condition or disease may provide the nurse an early warning laboratory test that leads to an effective intervention before inflammatory dysregulation can occur.

Summary

A person's predisposition for a greater or a lesser inflammatory response is determined by the interaction of genes and environment [9]. A dysregulated inflammatory response contributes to adverse outcomes in several illnesses in critically ill patients. Understanding normal, physiologic inflammation has progressed significantly with the advent of new and refined genomic technology. From traditional genetic associative studies, to transcriptome and proteomic investigations, researchers are increasing our understanding of the human response to irritants, injury, and infection by elucidating inflammatory signaling in health and disease. Findings from genomic studies are providing insight into clinical diagnosis and treatment of some of the most challenging acutely ill patients.

References

[1] Kumar VK, Fausto N, Abbas A. Robbins and Cotran pathologic basis of disease. 7th edition. Philadelphia: Saunders; 2005. p. 47, Chapter 2.

[2] Workman ML. The cellular basis of bacterial infection. Crit Care Nurs Clin North Am 2003;15:1–11.

[3] Sorenson TI, Nielson GG, Andersen PK, et al. Genetic and environmental influences on premature death in adult adoptees. N Engl J Med 1988;318: 727–32.

[4] Lashley FR. Clinical genetics in nursing practice. 3rd edition. New York: Springer; 2005.

[5] Majetschack M, Flohe S, Obertacke U, et al. Relation of a TNF gene polymorphism to severe sepsis in trauma patients. Ann Surg 1999;230:207–14.

[6] Tang GJ, Huang SL, Yien HW, et al. Tumor necrosis factor gene polymorphism and septic shock in surgical infection. Crit Care Med 2000;28:2733–6.

[7] Barber RC, Chang LY, Arnoldo BD, et al. Innate immunity SNPs are associated with risk for severe sepsis after burn injury. Clin Med Res 2006;4(4): 250–5.

[8] McDaniel DO, Hamilton J, Brock M, et al. Molecular analysis of inflammatory markers in trauma patients at risk of postinjury complications. J Trauma 2007;63(1):147–57.

[9] Stuber F, Klaschik S, Lehmann LE, et al. Cytokine promoter polymorphisms in severe sepsis. Clin Infect Dis 2005;41(Suppl 7):S416–20.

[10] Clark MF, Baudouin SV. A systematic review of the quality of genetic association studies in human sepsis. Intensive Care Med 2006;32:1706–12.

[11] McDunn JE, Chung TP, Laramie JM, et al. Physiologic genomics. Surgery 2006;139(2):133–9.

[12] van de Vijver MJ, He YD, van't Veer LJ, et al. A gene-expression signature as a predictor of survival in breast cancer. N Engl J Med 2002;347(25): 1999–2009.

[13] Sommers MS. The cellular basis of septic shock. Crit Care Nurs Clin North Am 2003;15(1):13–25.

[14] Hanash S. Proteomics. Nature 2003;22:226–32.

[15] Knight PR, Sreekumar AS, Siddiqui J, et al. Development of a sensitive microarray immunoassay and comparison with standard enzyme-linked immunoassay for cytokine analysis. Shock 2004;21:26–30.

[16] Chung TP, Laramie JM, Meyer DJ, et al. Molecular diagnostics in sepsis: from bench to bedside. J Am Coll Surg 2006;203:585–98.

[17] Prucha M, Moller E, Deogmer P, et al. Gene expression in septic patients manifests significant diagnostic signatures despite strong center-associated effects. Journal of Federation of European Biochemical Societies 2005;272(s1):AbstractA4. p. 49.

[18] MacGlashan D. Histamine: a mediator of inflammation. J Allergy Clin Immunol 2003;112(4 Suppl): S53–9.

[19] Ogawa Y, Calhoun WJ. The role of leukotrienes in airway inflammation. J Allergy Clin Immunol 2006;118(4):789–98.

[20] Frank MM. Hereditary angioedema: the clinical syndrome and its management in the United States. Immunol Allergy Clin North Am 2006;26(4): 653–68.

[21] Chaplin DD. Overview of the human immune response. J Allergy Clin Immunol 2006;117:S430–5.

[22] Morgan BP, Marchbank KJ, Longhi MP, et al. Complement: central to innate immunity and bridging to adaptive responses. Immunol Lett 2005;97: 171–9.

[23] Tosi MF. Innate immune responses to infection. J Allergy Clin Immunol 2005;116(2):241–9.

[24] Kapetanovic R, Cavaillon JM. Early events in innate immunity in the recognition of microbial pathogens. Expert Opin Biol Ther 2007;7(6):907–17.

[25] Short MA, Schlichting D, Qualy RL. From bench to bedside: a review of the clinical trial development plan of drotrecogin alfa (activated). Curr Med Res Opin 2006;22(12):2525–40.

[26] Hermans PWM, Hazelzet JA. Plasminogen activator inhibitor type 1 gene polymorphism and sepsis. Clin Infect Dis 2005;41:S453–8.

[27] Khanapure SP, Garvey DS, Janero D, et al. Eicosanoids in inflammation: biosynthesis, pharmacology, and therapeutic frontiers. Curr Top Med Chem 2007;7(3):311–40.

[28] Ogawa Y, Grant JA. Mediators of anaphylaxis. Immunol Allergy Clin North Am 2007;27(2): 249–60.

[29] Berger A. What are leukotrienes and how do they work in asthma? Br Med J 1999;319:90.

[30] Corwin EJ. Understanding cytokines part II: implications for nursing research and practice. Biol Res Nurs 2000b;2(1):41–8.

[31] Borish L, Steinke JW. Cytokines and chemokines. J Allergy Clin Immunol 2003;111(2 Suppl):S460–75.

[32] Rubinstein M, Dinarello CA, Oppenhiem JJ, et al. Recent advances in cytokine, cytokine receptors and signal transduction. Cytokine Growth Factor Rev 1998;9(2):175–81.

[33] Steinke JW, Borish L. Cytokines and chemokines. J Allergy Clin Immunol 2006;117(2):S441–5.

[34] Corwin EJ. Understanding cytokines part I: physiology and mechanism of action. Biol Res Nurs 2000a; 2(1):30–40.

[35] Giannoudis PV. Current concepts of the inflammatory response after major trauma: an update. Injury 2003;34(6):397–404.

[36] Papathanassoglou ED, Giannakopoulou MD, Bozas E. Genomic variations and susceptibility to sepsis. AACN Adv Crit Care 2006;17(4):394–422.

[37] Arcaroli J, Fessler MB, Abraham E. Genetic polymorphisms and sepsis. Shock 2005;24(4):300–12.

[38] Topel EJ, Smith J, Plow EF, et al. Genetic susceptibility to myocardial infarction and coronary artery disease. Hum Mol Genet 2006;15(Spec No 2): R117–23.

[39] Renner P, Roger T, Calandra T. Macrophage migration inhibitory factor: gene polymorphisms and susceptibility to inflammatory diseases. Clin Infect Dis 2005;41(Suppl 7):S513–9.

[40] Jawa RS, Kulaylat MN, Baumann H, et al. What is new in cytokine research related to trauma/critical care. Intensive Care Med 2006;21(2):63–85.

[41] Leaver SK, Finney SJ, Burke-Gaffney A, et al. Sepsis since the discovery of Toll-like receptors: disease concepts and therapeutic opportunities. Crit Care Med 2007;35(5):1404–10.

[42] Maizels RM, Yazdanbakhsh M. Immune regulation by helminth parasites: cellular and molecular mechanisms. Nat Rev Immunol 2003;3(9):733–44.

[43] Sepkowitz KA. Concentric circles and knockout mice: Advances in TB detection, diagnosis and treatment. In: The Medscape Journal, 2000. Available at: http://www.medscape.com/viewarticle/ 418771. Accessed August 24, 2007.

[44] NCBI. Molecular modeling: A method for unraveling protein structure and function. In: Just the Facts: A Basic Introduction to the Science Underlying NCBI Resources, 2004. Available at: http://www.ncbi.nlm. nih.gov/About/primer/molecularmod.html. Accessed September 1, 2007.

ELSEVIER
SAUNDERS

Crit Care Nurs Clin N Am 20 (2008) 223–231

CRITICAL CARE
NURSING CLINICS
OF NORTH AMERICA

Pharmacogenetics in Critical Care: Atrial Fibrillation as an Exemplar

Cynthia A. Prows, MSN, RN, FAAN[a],*,
Theresa A. Beery, PhD, RN, ACNP[b]

[a]Divisions of Patient Services and Human Genetics, Cincinnati Children's Hospital Medical Center,
3333 Burnet Avenue, Building E 5-249, ML 4006, Cincinnati, OH 45229-3039, USA
[b]College of Nursing, University of Cincinnati, 3110 Vine Street, Cincinnati, OH 45221-0038, USA

Every experienced clinician knows that variation in drug response between patients is the rule. In any setting, and in any situation, a person's response to medication is influenced by many different factors (Fig. 1) and bodily processes [1]. Examples of factors are the person's general health or existence of comorbidities, use of other medications or herbal products, body weight, and age. In critical care settings, confounding factors in drug response can be especially prevalent [2]. Bodily processes that influence medication response, referred to as pharmacokinetics, include absorption, distribution, metabolism, and elimination. Pharmacodynamics (what a drug does to the body) involves chemical interactions and receptor interactions [3]. Different proteins are involved in the various pharmacokinetic processes and pharmacodynamics interactions and each protein is encoded by a different gene.

These genes and their variant forms are the focus of pharmacogenetics/pharmacogenomics. Genes' variants that encode deficient, dysfunctional, or nonfunctioning proteins involved in medication processing can predispose a patient to unintended drug responses, either toxicity or inadequate efficacy [4,5]. Medication selection and dosing guided by pharmacogenetic (PG) test results and consideration of other environmental, health state, and lifestyle factors (see Fig. 1) are components of personalized medicine

[6,7]. PG testing can also be used after medication therapy has begun to determine if genetic factors are playing a role in a patient's unintended drug response.

This article uses atrial fibrillation as an exemplar to illustrate the purpose and challenges of using PG testing in critical care settings. With the expected growth in the number and applications of PG tests, nurses in critical care settings are likely to encounter patients whose care is being informed by PG test results. This article therefore also addresses relevant genetic/genomic competencies [8] for nurses when medication therapy is guided by PG testing.

Clinical scenario

A 68-year-old woman is 3 days post knee replacement surgery. She has developed new-onset atrial fibrillation (AF) and increased shortness of breath. Medical history includes:

Nonischemic heart failure, New York Heart Association (NYHA) class II with ejection fraction of 35%
Clinical depression
Osteoarthritis
Dyslipidemia

She states that she is upset because her doctor said she would have to take Coumadin. The patient reveals that her sister took Coumadin for AF and her health care providers never did get the dose right. Her sister suffered a major hemorrhagic stroke and died.

* Corresponding author.
E-mail address: cindy.prows@cchmc.org
(C.A. Prows).

0899-5885/08/$ - see front matter © 2008 Elsevier Inc. All rights reserved.
doi:10.1016/j.ccell.2008.01.006

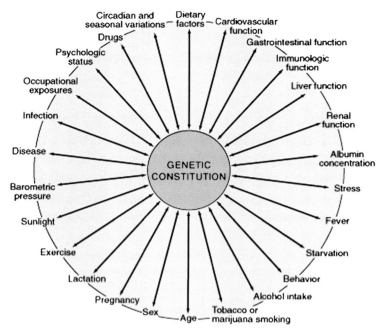

Fig. 1. Genetic, environmental, and developmental factors that can interact, causing variations in drug response among patients. (*From* Beers, MH, editor. The Merck manual of diagnosis and therapy. 18th edition. Whitehouse Station, NJ: Merck & Co., Inc.; 2006. Available at: http://www.merck.com/mmpe/. Accessed October 11, 2007; with permission.)

The patient received heparin until her international normalized ratio (INR) became therapeutic and Coumadin was started without initial bolus dosing. In addition to Coumadin, the patient was started on digoxin for heart rate control and naproxen for postoperative pain and inflammation. Previously prescribed medications that were continued during the hospitalization included:

Atorvastatin (for dyslipidemia)
Lisinopril (for heart failure)
Carvedilol (for heart failure)
Sertraline (Zoloft) (for clinical depression)
Furosemide as needed (for fluid retention)
Spironolactone (for heart failure)

Atrial fibrillation

AF affects more that 2.2 million Americans making it the most common sustained arrhythmia and the most frequent complication after cardiac surgery [9,10]. Although most cases of AF seem to be sporadic, mutations in genes encoding potassium channels and intercellular gap junctions can lead to heritable forms of AF [11–13]. In addition, renin-angiotensin system gene variants predispose to AF in the setting of elevated atrial pressure [14]. Not

only are genetic variants important in the origin of AF, but various polymorphisms can alter the patient response to the drugs used to treat it.

Atrial fibrillation treatment goals

The American College of Cardiology, the American Heart Association, and the European Society of Cardiology recommend heart rate control and antithrombotic therapy for patients who have AF [15]. Two major clinical trials (AF-FIRM and RACE) concluded that embolic events occur equally in patients treated by rate or rhythm control and there is no difference in quality of life and functional status; however, rate control is the preferred initial treatment for patients who have AF because both studies showed a decrease in primary endpoints with rate control [16,17].

Prevent thromboembolism

The most severe complications of AF include thromboembolism and stroke, so patient response to anticoagulants is of major interest to clinicians. The risk for stroke in people who have AF is two to three times that of the general population [18]. The timely administration and titration of anticoagulants can prevent or mitigate these life-threatening events [19]. The concomitant heart failure in the patient described in the case study increases her risk for thromboembolism even with new-onset AF. In such situations, evidence-based guidelines recommend a vitamin K antagonist, such as warfarin, for anticoagulation therapy [15].

Control heart rate

Patients who have AF often require medication to slow the ventricular response. For rate control in people who have permanent sustained AF either nondihydropyridine calcium channel antagonists (verapamil, diltiazem) or beta-blockers (esmolol, metoprolol, propanolol) are recommended. For patients who do not have pre-excitation, digoxin or amiodarone is recommended for rate control [15]. Amiodarone is one of a wide variety of drugs that can prolong the QT interval in people at genetic risk, creating a vulnerability to the potentially lethal ventricular arrhythmia, torsade de pointes. Subsequent hemodynamic compromise is seen clinically as syncope or sudden cardiac death.

Genetic testing for warfarin response

Safely and effectively dosing warfarin continues to be a challenge to prescribers despite the drug's having been approved by the US Food and Drug Administration (FDA) more than 50 years ago [7]. Warfarin has a narrow therapeutic range with significant interindividual dose–response variability with a consequence of life-threatening bleeding episodes if overdosed. The target range for prothrombin time expressed as an INR is 2.0 to 3.0, with a target of 2.5 [20]. Even after considering known factors that contribute to variability, such as age, weight, concomitant medications, diet, alcohol consumption, and comorbidities, considerable interindividual dose–response variability remains [21–23]. There are many different genes that encode proteins involved in warfarin response and polymorphisms in several of the genes are associated with much of the remaining dose–response variability [24]. This section discusses the two primary genes for which genetic testing is commercially available to identify patients who need lower or, in some cases, higher doses of warfarin than would normally be calculated after consideration of nongenetic factors alone.

CYP2C9

CYP2C9 enzyme is important for warfarin metabolism. Specifically, warfarin is a 50:50 racemic mixture of S-warfarin and R-warfarin. S-warfarin is three to five times as potent as R-warfarin. CYP2C9 is the principle enzyme that metabolizes S-warfarin to its two inactive components. CYP2C9 is not involved in the metabolism of R-warfarin [25,26].

The *CYP2C9* gene is part of a family of 57 different genes called cytochrome P450 (CYP). Each gene in this family produces a different isoenzyme. As a family, these enzymes metabolize/detoxify exogenous materials, such as drugs and environmental chemicals. They also metabolize endogenous materials, such as bile acids, retinoids, and saturated and unsaturated fatty acids [27].

CYP2C9 has more than 30 variant forms (alleles) but not all change the amount or function of the resulting enzyme [28]. Many clinical studies demonstrated the relationship between *CYP2C9* variants and warfarin dose. Specifically, the studies looked for associations with *CYP2C9*1* (wild-type allele or "normal" allele) and the two most common variants, *CYP2C9*2* and *CYP2C9*3*. (For a review of these studies, see Ref. [26]). *CYP2C9*2* and *CYP2C9*3* have been shown to reduce the metabolism of warfarin by 30% to 50% and around 90%, respectively [22]. These are the alleles most commonly analyzed in commercial laboratories that provide PG testing.

Gage and colleagues [21] measured the contribution to warfarin dose variability of *CYP2C9* genotype status and many of the nongenetic factors. The investigators found that about 28% of maintenance dose variability could be attributed to the assessed nongenetic factors, whereas *CYP2C9* variants attributed to 10% of the dose variability. *CYP2C9* therefore only partly explains the genetic variability in required doses.

VKORC1

Warfarin's action is directed at the enzyme, vitamin K epoxide reductase (VKOR) [29,30]. VKOR is necessary for activating vitamin K–dependent clotting factors (II, VII, IX, X) involved in thrombin formation. The VKOR complex subunit 1 (*VKORC1*) gene produces the primary protein component of VKOR [31,32]. Five common *VKORC1* variants associated with either high or low warfarin dose requirements have been described [33].

Several studies have compared the contributions of *VKORC1* variants and *CYP2C9* variants to warfarin dose requirements. *VKORC1* variants explained about 15% [34] to 30% [33] of interindividual variability, whereas *CYP2C9* explained about 10% [33] to 18% [34] of the variability in warfarin maintenance dose. Other investigators found that *CYP2C9* genotype accounted for about a sixfold difference in dose between patients, whereas a twofold difference in warfarin dose was attributed to *VKORC1* genotype [35]. These aforementioned studies were done primarily in whites of European or Israeli descent. Further studies have demonstrated that the presence and frequency of *VKORC1* and *CYP2C9* variants and the magnitude of their effects can differ between populations [36,37].

Clinical scenario (continued)

A warfarin PG test was ordered on the same day the AF was diagnosed. Within 48 hours, the prescriber received results that the patient's CYP2C9 genotype predicted a poor metabolizer phenotype and her VKORC1 genotype predicted a warfarin-sensitive phenotype. Similar to her sister, therefore, the patient's genotype predisposes her to the bleeding risks associated with warfarin.

Pharmacogenetic testing for warfarin in clinical settings

Based on the evidence of warfarin high/low dose requirements associated with *VKORC1* and *CYP2C9* variants, an advisory committee of the FDA voted in favor of relabeling warfarin to include genomic and test information [38]. A working paper available at the AEI Brookings Joint Center for Regulatory Studies Web site (http://www.aei-brookings.org/publications/index.php?tab=types&typeid=8; accessed July 30, 2007) estimates that 85,000 serious bleeding episodes and 17,000 strokes could be avoided annually by routinely using genetic testing to guide warfarin therapy [39]. Despite these high level organizational supports for warfarin PG testing, it is still not clear how prescribers are to factor in genotype information together with age, weight, comorbidities, and other environmental factors, such as diet, alcohol consumption, and concomitant medications, to determine a dose for a specific patient [40].

In the clinical scenario, prescribers received the patient's genotype and predicted phenotype results within 48 hours. A 2-day business turnaround time for PG test results is customary for the Cincinnati Children's Hospital Medical Center. Turnaround time can be expected to decrease with continual advances in molecular diagnostic technology [41].

Although it would be ideal to delay warfarin initiation until results are available, this is not necessary. Results received within 2 days of initiation can still inform the provider whether a cautious or more aggressive approach to dose changes may be needed. Knowing that the patient in the case scenario has a genetic predisposition to warfarin sensitivity, prescribers would be prudent to use extra caution in the rate of dose increases and the number of INRs obtained during the warfarin initiation period. Nurses informed of the genetic predisposition would know to be especially diligent at assessing for signs of bleeding and teaching the patient to do the same. Genetic testing for warfarin dose response would be clinically more useful if actual initiation and maintenance doses could be predicted.

In response to clinicians' need for warfarin therapy decision support, several groups of investigators have identified sensitive genetic and nongenetic factors for use in dosing algorithms [21,24,42,43]. Prospective clinical outcome studies evaluating the use of various dosing algorithms are underway. The results of these studies will be especially important now that the warfarin label has been updated by the FDA to include information about the role of *CYP2C9* and *VKORC1* variations in dose response and the commercial availability of tests for these genes [44]. On the FDA Web site, a question-and-answer fact sheet about the new labeling states, "Healthcare professionals might incorporate the genetic information on *CYP2C9* and *VKORC1*, along with various clinical considerations and patient characteristics (eg, age, body weight) to better estimate the initial warfarin doses for patients" (http://www.fda.gov/cder/drug/infopage/warfarin/qa.htm; accessed August 30, 2007). In light of this, nurses working in anticoagulation clinics and critical care settings can expect to see an increased use of genetic testing in patients who require warfarin therapy.

Concomitant medications and warfarin response

The 68-year-old woman described in the clinical scenario was on medications that, independent of the patient's genetic predisposition, could potentially moderate warfarin response: naproxen, sertraline, and spironolactone. It is important to consider whether or not concomitant medications are likely to change during warfarin therapy. For instance, the naproxen was prescribed to treat postoperative pain and inflammation and would be discontinued when the indications resolve.

Sertraline and spironolactone would likely be administered on a more long-term basis.

Naproxen can potentially have a major interaction with warfarin that can increase the risk for bleeding [45]. It can be used along with warfarin as long as INRs and prothrombin times are closely monitored. In this clinical scenario, warfarin therapy was initiated at the time naproxen was coadministered. When naproxen is discontinued, close monitoring of INRs is important and warfarin dose adjustments may be necessary.

The Micromedex Healthcare Series [45] lists sertraline and spironolactone as potentially having moderate interactions with warfarin. Sertraline can increase the risk for bleeding, whereas spironolactone can decrease the anticoagulant effectiveness of warfarin. Unlike naproxen, these two medications are likely to be prescribed on a long-term basis for the 68-year-old woman. The effects of these medications on INR are factors in the initiation period and are likely to continue during the maintenance period. Any changes in dosing or a cessation of one or both of these medications during warfarin therapy requires close monitoring of INRs and warfarin dose adjustments may be necessary.

Genetic influence on heart rate control medication response

The genes and their variants associated with unintended drug response for heart rate control medications are not as well studied as the two aforementioned variant genes associated with warfarin response. The patient described earlier in this article was placed on digoxin for rate control. Bioavailability and clearance of digoxin can vary widely resulting in differing plasma drug levels from person to person despite the same dose. P-glycoprotein (Pg-p), the product of the multidrug-resistance 1/ATP-binding cassette, subfamily B (*MDR1/ABCB1*) gene (http://www.ihop-net.org/UniPub/iHOP/bng/90987.html; accessed September 3, 2007) is a transmembrane transporter [46]. One common polymorphism (C3435T) in *MDR1* has been associated with reduced duodenal expression of Pg-p and significantly higher digoxin plasma levels [47]. Other studies demonstrate lower apparent digoxin volume of distribution [48] or clinically insignificant differences in digoxin concentrations in subjects homozygous for the polymorphism, however [49]. Further investigations are therefore needed before this gene can be used in clinical settings for PG testing purposes.

As mentioned earlier, other rate-control medications may be used for patients who have AF. Most beta-blockers, including S-metoprolol, carvedilol, and propanolol, are metabolized by *CYP2D6* [28]. Most laboratories that provide PG testing offer *CYP2D6* genotyping. Combinations of *CYP2D6* alleles can result in four possible phenotypes: poor metabolizer (PM), intermediate metabolizer (IM), extensive metabolizer (EM), and ultra-rapid metabolizer (UM) [50,51]. PM phenotype is associated with a combination of two alleles that either do not produce enzyme or produce nonfunctional enzyme. IM phenotype is associated with a combination of two alleles that produce deficient enzyme. EM phenotype is also referred to as the "normal metabolizer" and is associated with a combination of two common alleles that produce the expected amount of enzyme activity. People who have three or more copies of the alleles that produce normal *CYP2D6* enzyme are genetically predisposed to UM phenotype because they produce higher levels of *CYP2D6* enzyme activity than EMs [52].

Of all the beta-blockers metabolized by *CYP2D6*, metoprolol is the most dependent, with 70% to 80% of its metabolism reliant on *CYP2D6* [53]. Higher metoprolol plasma concentrations have been detected in PMs [54,55] but differences in clinical outcomes when comparing PMs with EMs have not been consistent [53]. Recent prospective studies did not find statistically significant increased adverse effects in *CYP2D6* poor metabolizers despite having higher plasma concentrations [54,56]. One study of healthy adults given a single dose of metoprolol did demonstrate that UMs had dramatically lower plasma concentrations of metoprolol and statistically higher heart rate than EMs. There were no differences in blood pressure response to the drug, however [52].

Another gene that has received extensive attention in studies investigating beta-blocker response is beta-1 adrenergic receptor gene (ADRB1). For a comprehensive review of existing studies, see Shin and Johnson [53]. The authors concluded that although the specific polymorphism, Arg389Gly, repeatedly shows clinical effect, there are many other genes involved in a person's response to beta-blockers that need further study before any particular beta-blocker–related PG test can be routinely used in clinical practice.

Before and during her hospital stay, the 68-year-old woman in the clinical scenario had been on a nonselective alpha- and beta-blocker, carvedilol, and then digoxin was added during the hospitalization, which is not uncommon [57]. Carvedilol is primarily metabolized by *CYP2D6* and *CYP2C9* [45]. Although gene tests for these enzymes are commercially available, studies measuring the amount of drug response variability attributed by these genes in patients still need to be done.

Concomitant medications and rate control medication response

The patient in the clinical scenario was on medications known to interact with one another. Carvedilol and atorvastatin have been shown to each increase digoxin levels by up to 20% [58,59]; therefore, digoxin levels need to be monitored and nurses need to carefully assess for any signs of digoxin toxicity (nausea, vomiting, cardiac arrhythmias). Digoxin has a secondary role in heart failure treatment for patients who have atrial fibrillation or those who are symptomatic on all other usual drugs. Increased blood pressure can occur when nonsteroidal antiinflammatory drugs (NSAIDs) and β-adrenergic blockers are taken together [45]. When concurrent therapy is required, as in the clinical scenario, nurses need to monitor and document the patient's blood pressure carefully so that dosage adjustment for the beta-blockers can be made. Lisinopril is an angiotensin-converting enzyme that lowers aldosterone levels and can cause hyperkalemia when taken concurrently with potassium-sparing diuretics, such as spironolactone [45].

Implications for nursing practice: genetics and genomics essentials

A consensus panel of leaders from nearly 50 organizations have published *Essential Nursing Competencies and Curricula Guidelines for Genetics and Genomics* [8]. Forty-seven organizations endorsed the document by the time it was published. Some of those endorsing organizations that have members who work in critical care include the Academy of Medical-Surgical Nurses, the American Academy of Nurses, the American Nurses Association, the American Association of Neuroscience Nurses, the Council of Cardiovascular Nursing of the American Heart Association, Sigma Theta Tau International, and the Society of Vascular Nursing.

The competency document describes the minimal genetic/genomic competencies for all registered nurses, regardless of level of academic preparation, practice setting, or specialty. The competencies are organized within two main categories: professional responsibilities and professional practice domain. Within the professional practice domain, competencies are divided between nursing assessment; identification; referral activities; and provision of education, care, and support [8]. A selection of the competencies is used to frame the discussion for nursing implications of using pharmacogenetics in critical care settings.

Provides clients with credible, accurate, appropriate, and current genetic and genomic information, resources, services, and/or technologies that facilitate decision making [8]. In a critical care setting, it may not be feasible to involve patients in the decision-making process regarding PG testing if their cognitive abilities are impaired because of disease, injury, or medication. The nurse may therefore need to give information about any prescribed PG test to a family member or professional who is making health care decisions on behalf of the patient. Information should include the purpose and limitations of the test. Patients or their advocates need to understand that PG test results provide additional information that can help prescribers select or adjust medication doses to reduce the risk for adverse drug reactions and improve the chances of achieving therapeutic targets in a timely fashion. In some cases PG test results may help prescribers choose the medication most likely to achieve the desired therapeutic effect. Because gene variants are just one type of factor that impacts on drug response, however, careful patient monitoring is still required and assurance of problem-free medication therapy cannot be given. Patients or their advocates also need to understand that PG test results may not be relevant for all medications needed to treat the patient. Finally, depending on the type of analysis performed in the laboratory, a negative or normal test result may be a false negative if all possible variants associated with altered gene function were not analyzed.

The way in which a nurse conveys this information depends on his or her knowledge, access to resources, and the accommodations within the critical care environment for this type of patient/advocate teaching. Nurses who are knowledgeable about PG testing are able to discuss the benefits and limitations of the test. In a critical care setting, however, finding the time and a quiet environment conducive for this type of discussion can be elusive. When giving the patient/advocate written information it is helpful to first briefly overview its content and assess the patient/advocate's reading ability. Reading material allows the patient/advocate to focus on the information at a time that is convenient for him or her and frees the nurse to respond to questions.

Provides clients with interpretation of selective genetic and genomic information or services; assesses clients' knowledge, perceptions, and response to genetic and genomic information [8]. Oftentimes the initial explanation about what the PG test results mean for the patient's plan of care is provided by the advanced practice nurse or physician who ordered the test. The critical care nurse at the bedside has the important role of following up with the patients/advocates to make sure they understood the information that was presented, clarify any misunderstandings, and address any concerns the patients/families express regarding the subsequent plan of care. Two important points that differentiate genetic test results from other types of laboratory results include: genetic test results may be relevant to a patient's future health care because inherited genes, for the most part, do not change; and a patient's genetic test result may be relevant to biologic family members because they share inherited genes.

Evaluates impact and effectiveness of genetic and genomic technology, information, interventions, and treatments on clients' outcome. Critical care nurses have a key role in evaluating the effectiveness of PG-guided medication therapy. As is the case for all treatments and therapies provided to the patient, it is the nurse who consistently monitors the patient for clinical improvement and closely assesses for early signs of drug toxicity. When patients/advocates receive information about PG tests, it is within the nurse's role to evaluate the effectiveness of the presented information, whether that is in verbal, written, or electronic format.

Summary

PG testing is currently not routine in critical care settings but the recent FDA changes in the warfarin label are likely to lead to critical care nurses encountering physician or nurse practitioner orders for such testing. Although the science for pharmacogenetics is complex, the components of patient teaching are not beyond that which nurses already provide about other laboratory, disease, and treatment-based information. Nurses need to keep in mind that PG test results do not replace the need to consider other factors when anticipating and monitoring a patient's response to one or more medications. It is reasonable to expect, however, that as the science of pharmacogenetics and pharmacogenomics expands and discoveries are translated in clinical settings, the additional information from PG test results will help prescribers select or adjust medication doses to reduce the risk for adverse drug reactions and improve the chances of achieving therapeutic targets in a timely fashion.

References

[1] Leeder JS. Pharmacogenetics and pharmacogenomics. Pediatr Clin North Am 2001;48(3):765–81.
[2] Freeman BD, McLeod HL. Challenges of implementing pharmacogenetics in the critical care environment. Nat Rev Drug Discov 2004;3(1):88–93.
[3] Porter RS, Kaplan JL. Merck manuals online medical library for healthcare professionals. Whitehouse Station (NJ): Merck Research Laboratories; 2006–2007. Available at: http://www.merck.com/mmpe/index.html. Accessed October 11, 2007.
[4] Evans WE, McLeod HL. Pharmacogenomics—drug disposition, drug targets, and side effects. N Engl J Med 2003;348(6):538–49.
[5] Weinshilboum R, Wang L. Pharmacogenomics: bench to bedside. Nat Rev Drug Discov 2004;3(9):739–48.
[6] Woodcock J. The prospects for "personalized medicine" in drug development and drug therapy. Clin Pharmacol Ther 2007;81(2):164–9.
[7] Lesko LJ. Personalized medicine: elusive dream or imminent reality? Clin Pharmacol Ther 2007;81(6):807–16.
[8] Consensus Panel on Genetic/Genomic Nursing Competencies. Essential nursing competencies and curricula guidelines for genetics and genomics. Silver Spring (MD): American Nurses Association; 2006.
[9] Go AS, Hylek EM, Phillips KA, et al. Prevalence of diagnosed atrial fibrillation in adults: national implications for rhythm management and stroke prevention: the AnTicoagulation and Risk Factors in Atrial Fibrillation (ATRIA) Study. JAMA 2001;285(18):2370–5.
[10] Motsinger AA, Donahue BS, Brown NJ, et al. Risk factor interactions and genetic effects associated with post-operative atrial fibrillation. Pac Symp Biocomput 2006;11:584–95.
[11] Lai LP, Su MJ, Yeh HM, et al. Association of the human minK gene 38G allele with atrial fibrillation: evidence of possible genetic control on the pathogenesis of atrial fibrillation. Am Heart J 2002;144(3):485–90.
[12] Chen YH, Xu SJ, Bendahhou S, et al. KCNQ1 gain-of-function mutation in familial atrial fibrillation. Science 2003;299(5604):251–4.

[13] Firouzi M, Ramanna H, Kok B, et al. Association of human connexin40 gene polymorphisms with atrial vulnerability as a risk factor for idiopathic atrial fibrillation. Circ Res 2004;95(4):e29–33.

[14] Tsai CT, Lai LP, Lin JL, et al. Renin-angiotensin system gene polymorphisms and atrial fibrillation. Circulation 2004;109(13):1640–6.

[15] Fuster V, Ryden LE, Cannom DS, et al. ACC/AHA/ ESC 2006 guidelines for the management of patients with atrial fibrillation—executive summary: a report of the American College of Cardiology/American Heart Association Task Force on Practice Guide-lines and the European Society of Cardiology Committee for Practice Guidelines (Writing Committee to Revise the 2001 Guidelines for the Management of Patients With Atrial Fibrillation). J Am Coll Cardiol 2006;48(4):854–906.

[16] Snow V, Weiss KB, LeFevre M, et al. Management of newly detected atrial fibrillation: a clinical practice guideline from the American Academy of Family Physicians and the American College of Physicians. Ann Intern Med 2003;139(12):1009–17.

[17] McNamara RL, Tamariz LJ, Segal JB, et al. Man-agement of atrial fibrillation: review of the evidence for the role of pharmacologic therapy, electrical cardioversion, and echocardiography. Ann Intern Med 2003;139(12):1018–33.

[18] Frost L, Engholm G, Johnsen S, et al. Incident stroke after discharge from the hospital with a diag-nosis of atrial fibrillation. Am J Med 2000;108(1): 36–40.

[19] Roepke TK, Abbott GW. Pharmacogenetics and cardiac ion channels. Vascul Pharmacol 2006;44(2): 90–106.

[20] Hirsh J, Fuster V, Ansell J, et al. American Heart Association/American College of Cardiology Foun-dation guide to warfarin therapy. J Am Coll Cardiol 2003;41(9):1633–52.

[21] Gage BF, Eby C, Milligan PE, et al. Use of pharma-cogenetics and clinical factors to predict the mainte-nance dose of warfarin. Thromb Haemost 2004; 91(1):87–94.

[22] Sanderson S, Emery J, Higgins J. CYP2C9 gene variants, drug dose, and bleeding risk in warfarin-treated patients: a HuGEnet systematic review and meta-analysis. Genet Med 2005;7(2):97–104.

[23] Bristol-Myers Squibb Company: Medication Guide: Coumadin (COU-ma-din) tablets, (warfarin sodium tablets, USP) crystalline. Princeton (NJ): Bristol-Myers Squibb Company; 2006 patient information. Available at: http://www.fda.gov/ cder/Offices/ODS/MG/warfarinMG.pdf. Accessed October 11, 2007.

[24] Wadelius M, Chen LY, Eriksson N, et al. Associa-tion of warfarin dose with genes involved in its action and metabolism. Hum Genet 2007;121(1): 23–34.

[25] Aithal GP, Day CP, Kesteven PJ, et al. Association of polymorphisms in the cytochrome P450 CYP2C9

with warfarin dose requirement and risk of bleeding complications. Lancet 1999;353(9154):717–9.

[26] Daly AK, King BP. Pharmacogenetics of oral anti-coagulants. Pharmacogenetics 2003;13(5):247–52.

[27] Nebert DW, Russell DW. Clinical importance of the cytochromes P450. Lancet 2002;360(9340):1155–62.

[28] Flockhart DA. Drug interaction table (cytochrome P450 system). Available at: http://medicine.iupui. edu/flockhart/. Accessed October 11, 2007.

[29] Bell RG, Matschiner JT. Warfarin and the inhibition of vitamin K activity by an oxide metabolite. Nature 1972;237(5349):32–3.

[30] Bell RG, Sadowski JA, Matschiner JT. Mechanism of action of warfarin. Warfarin and metabolism of vitamin K 1. Biochemistry 1972;11(10):1959–61.

[31] Rost S, Fregin A, Ivaskevicius V, et al. Mutations in VKORC1 cause warfarin resistance and multiple coagulation factor deficiency type 2. Nature 2004; 427(6974):537–41.

[32] Li T, Chang CY, Jin DY, et al. Identification of the gene for vitamin K epoxide reductase. Nature 2004; 427(6974):541–4.

[33] Wadelius M, Chen LY, Downes K, et al. Common VKORC1 and GGCX polymorphisms associated with warfarin dose. Pharmacogenomics J 2005; 5(4):262–70.

[34] Carlquist JF, Horne BD, Muhlestein JB, et al. Geno-types of the cytochrome p450 isoform, CYP2C9, and the vitamin K epoxide reductase complex subunit 1 conjointly determine stable warfarin dose: a pro-spective study. J Thromb Thrombolysis 2006;22(3): 191–7.

[35] Hamberg AK, Dahl ML, Barban M, et al. A PK-PD model for predicting the impact of age, CYP2C9, and VKORC1 genotype on individualization of warfarin therapy. Clin Pharmacol Ther 2007;81(4): 529–38.

[36] Takahashi H, Wilkinson GR, Nutescu EA, et al. Different contributions of polymorphisms in VKORC1 and CYP2C9 to intra- and inter-popula-tion differences in maintenance dose of warfarin in Japanese, Caucasians and African-Americans. Pharmacogenet Genomics 2006;16(2):101–10.

[37] Kimura R, Miyashita K, Kokubo Y, et al. Geno-types of vitamin K epoxide reductase, gamma-glutamyl carboxylase, and cytochrome P450 2C9 as determinants of daily warfarin dose in Japanese patients. Thromb Res 2007;120(2):181–6.

[38] Food and Drug Administration. Guidance for industry: pharmacogenomic data submissions. Rockville (MD): US Food and Drug Administra-tion; 2005. p. 28.

[39] McWilliam A, Lutter R, Nardinelli C. Health care savings from personalizing medicine using genetic testing: the case of warfarin. Washington (DC): AEI-Brookings Joint Center for Regulatory Studies; 2006.

[40] McClain MR, Palomaki GE, Piper M, et al. A rapid ACCE Review of CYP2C9 and VKORC1 allele

testing to inform warfarin dosing in adults at elevated risk for thrombotic events to avoid serious bleeding. Providence (RI): Women & Infants Hospital; 2007. p. 74.

[41] Tsongalis GJ. DNA STAT: the ability to perform clinical analysis in real time. Expert Rev Mol Diagn 2005;5(5):627–8.

[42] Sconce EA, Khan TI, Wynne HA, et al. The impact of CYP2C9 and VKORC1 genetic polymorphism and patient characteristics upon warfarin dose requirements: proposal for a new dosing regimen. Blood 2005;106(7):2329–33.

[43] Millican EA, Lenzini PA, Milligan PE, et al. Genetic-based dosing in orthopedic patients beginning warfarin therapy. Blood 2007;110(5):1511–5.

[44] Ray T. FDA updates warfarin label to explain genetic links to response; says change not meant as 'directive' for doctors. GenomeWeb Daily News 2007. Available at: http://www.genomeweb.com/issues/news/141730-1.html. Accessed October 11, 2007.

[45] Thomson Healthcare. Micromedex healthcare series, vol 2007. Greenwood (CO): Thomson Healthcare, Inc.; 2007. Available at: http://mcmicromed1/hcs/librarian/PFPUI/4aY1JnAY24tr8em. Accessed September 24, 2007.

[46] Kimchi-Sarfaty C, Marple AH, Shinar S, et al. Ethnicity-related polymorphisms and haplotypes in the human ABCB1 gene. Pharmacogenomics 2007; 8(1):29–39.

[47] Hoffmeyer S, Burk O, von Richter O, et al. Functional polymorphisms of the human multidrug-resistance gene: multiple sequence variations and correlation of one allele with P-glycoprotein expression and activity in vivo. Proc Natl Acad Sci U S A 2000;97(7):3473–8.

[48] Comets E, Verstuyft C, Lavielle M, et al. Modelling the influence of MDR1 polymorphism on digoxin pharmacokinetic parameters. Eur J Clin Pharmacol 2007;63(5):437–49.

[49] Kurzawski M, Bartnicka L, Florczak M, et al. Impact of ABCB1 (MDR1) gene polymorphism and P-glycoprotein inhibitors on digoxin serum concentration in congestive heart failure patients. Pharmacol Rep 2007;59(1):107–11.

[50] Sistonen J, Sajantila A, Lao O, et al. CYP2D6 worldwide genetic variation shows high frequency of altered activity variants and no continental structure. Pharmacogenet Genomics 2007;17(2):93–101.

[51] Zanger UM, Fischer J, Raimundo S, et al. Comprehensive analysis of the genetic factors determining expression and function of hepatic CYP2D6. Pharmacogenetics 2001;11(7):573–85.

[52] Kirchheiner J, Heesch C, Bauer S, et al. Impact of the ultrarapid metabolizer genotype of cytochrome P450 2D6 on metoprolol pharmacokinetics and pharmacodynamics. Clin Pharmacol Ther 2004;76(4):302–12.

[53] Shin J, Johnson JA. Pharmacogenetics of beta-blockers. Pharmacotherapy 2007;27(6):874–87.

[54] Zineh I, Beitelshees AL, Gaedigk A, et al. Pharmacokinetics and CYP2D6 genotypes do not predict metoprolol adverse events or efficacy in hypertension. Clin Pharmacol Ther 2004;76(6):536–44.

[55] Ismail R, Teh LK. The relevance of CYP2D6 genetic polymorphism on chronic metoprolol therapy in cardiovascular patients. J Clin Pharm Ther 2006; 31(1):99–109.

[56] Fux R, Morike K, Prohmer AM, et al. Impact of CYP2D6 genotype on adverse effects during treatment with metoprolol: a prospective clinical study. Clin Pharmacol Ther 2005;78(4):378–87.

[57] Taccetta-Chapnick M. Using carvedilol to treat heart failure. Crit Care Nurse 2002;22(2):36–40 42–46, 48 passim.

[58] Wermeling DP, Field CJ, Smith DA, et al. Effects of long-term oral carvedilol on the steady-state pharmacokinetics of oral digoxin in patients with mild to moderate hypertension. Pharmacotherapy 1994;14(5):600–6.

[59] Boyd RA, Stern RH, Stewart BH, et al. Atorvastatin coadministration may increase digoxin concentrations by inhibition of intestinal P-glycoprotein-mediated secretion. J Clin Pharmacol 2000;40(1): 91–8.

ELSEVIER
SAUNDERS

CRITICAL CARE
NURSING CLINICS
OF NORTH AMERICA

Crit Care Nurs Clin N Am 20 (2008) 233–237

Neonatal Genetic Testing is More Than Screening

Carole Kenner, DNS, RNC, FAAN[a,b,*],
Judith A. Lewis, PhD, RNC, FAAN[c], Jana L. Pressler, PhD, RN[b],
Cindy M. Little, PhD, RNC[d]

[a]Council of International Neonatal Nurses (COINN), 708 Capri Place, Edmond, OK 73034, USA
[b]College of Nursing, University of Oklahoma, 1100 North Stonewall Avenue, Oklahoma City, OK 73117, USA
[c]School of Nursing, Virginia Commonwealth University, 1100 East Leigh Street, Richmond, VA 23219, USA
[d]Old Dominion University, Technology Building, Room 357D, Norfolk, VA, USA

The ability to identify presymptomatically a disease or the future risk for a disease seems wonderful on the surface—but is it? This article explores what constitutes newborn genetic testing, the use of the family history tool in assessments, and the ethical and legal dilemmas arising from scientific genetic and technology breakthroughs.

Newborn screening

Screening tests provide for the early identification of children having various disorders or who are at increased risk for experiencing subsequent disorders [1]. Historically newborn screening tests have been relatively simple, inexpensive tests that are completed to determine whether or not an infant is in need of further diagnostics, examination, or special care [2]. Examples of such screening tests include postnatal tests (eg, Apgar [3–6], Postnatal Complications Scale [7]; Parmalee, 1974, unpublished manuscript), developmental tests (Denver Developmental Screening Test [8,9], Infant Motor Scale [10,11]), and medical tests for certain disorders. In the article that follows, the screening tests discussed focus exclusively on medical screening tests.

Historical overview

In the early 1960s Dr. Robert Guthrie developed a blood test for phenylketonuria (PKU), a metabolic disorder that results in developmental delays and mental retardation. This blood test revolutionized the diagnosis of PKU and its treatment. Before the Guthrie test, PKU was not determined until developmental delays were apparent and often irreversible nervous system damage was done. Early detection results in generally a better quality of life and fewer complications. It is doubtful that anyone would question the need for or the ethics of this test. Other conditions for which testing is done are not that clear-cut, however. With the advent of tandem mass spectrometry (MS/MS) more than a decade ago and the completion of the human genome mapping identifying the approximate placement of 22,000 genes on the 23 pairs of chromosomes, the possibility of prenatal or even preconceptual testing for predisposition for diseases became possible [12].

Approximately 4.1 million newborns are tested annually in the United States under the guise of newborn medical screening. Such medical screening is mandated by every state in the United States. The exact medical screening tests required for newborns vary from state to state, however. Some states require only 4 tests, whereas other require more than 40. For example, the state of Oklahoma requires seven medical tests:

Congenital hypothyroid
Congenital adrenal hyperplasia

* Corresponding author. University of Oklahoma College of Nursing, Suite 116, 1100 North Stonewall, Oklahoma City, OK 73117.

  E-mail address: carole-kenner@ouhsc.edu (C. Kenner).

Phenylketonuria (PKU)

Hemoglobinopathies, including sickle cell anemia and thalassemia

Transferase-deficient galactosemia

Cystic fibrosis

Medium chain acyl-CoA dehydrogenase [13]

The Associated Press reported in the *The Oklahoman*, July 15, 2007, that since 2004, when there was a push toward more aggressive comprehensive screening, the rate of babies tested has gone from 38% to 87.5%. There are no national guidelines; therefore, these data are accurate only in the states that are most aggressive in their screening efforts. The National Newborn Screening and Genetics Resource Center (http://genes-r-us.uths casa.edu/) provides a complete list by state of these test requirements. With technological advances, such as mass tandem spectrometry, only a small amount of blood is needed to run multiple tests [14]. These tests are minimally invasive or noninvasive. So what is the problem? Should we want to know about all problems that exist? Not all conditions that are found are treatable. Just because we can run a certain screening test, should we?

Commercial enterprises have entered into the business of genetic testing. For example, Pediatrix Screening offers StepOne, a screening service that determines a baby's risk for more than 50 inherited disorders through a simple procedure. (http://www.pediatrix.com/body_screening.cfm?id= 222&oTopID=94). Other companies offer DNA, RNA, or protein analysis for specific diseases with the marketing aspect focusing on predicting future problems. These tests are being marketed directly to the consumer with little information on the gamut of diseases that it tests or the prognosis for the conditions. No actual regulation of this industry exists. *A Brief Primer on Genetic Testing* is available on the Human Genome Web site at http://www.genome.gov/10506784 to provide accurate information to health professionals and the patients and families they serve. The Newborn Screening Act Sheets give algorithms for diagnosis and treatment (http://www.acmg. net/resources/policies/ACT/condition-analyte-links. htm). This approach may not be bad, because involving the consumer and transparency of health care are part of the Institute of Medicine's quality and safety series that was started in 1999. The catch is that the practice of medical screening and testing of newborns is virtually unregulated.

The testing dilemmas

Newborn screening programs, as they were originally called, have evolved to having an emphasis on genetic conditions, including newborn hearing. But these tests and their numbers vary from state to state and fall under the aegis of state health departments. Each state exercises autonomy in deciding which conditions to track, whether or how to obtain written informed consent from the parents, how to record and report results, and follow-up mechanisms for results that are determined by the state to be of concern [15]. The challenge is compounded when the laboratory that runs the test uses technology that screens for more conditions than included in that state's screening program and reports a positive screen for a condition not covered by that state's mandated follow-up program.

A similar situation could arise when a child is born in a state that is not the same as the state of the parent's residence. If, for example, a mother delivers in a perinatal center across the state border from her residence, the screening performed by the hospital may be for a panel of conditions that differs from those screened for in the parent's home state. As a consequence, it is possible that a newborn may be screened for conditions for which there is no follow-up in the state of residence but may not be screened for conditions mandated for screening by the home state.

These issues could be resolved if there were national guidelines for newborn screening and a standardized testing service. There have been recommendations toward this goal and the disparities among states have decreased. Although the American College of Medical Genetics reviewed the scientific literature and recommended such policies, including universal screening for 29 core conditions in 2005 [16], the lack of universal access to a consensus and evidence-based set of universal screening guidelines has not been a national priority. Part of this delay in promoting national regulation comes from the governmental stance of state purview of oversight. Another part of the equation is the concern over ethical and potentially legal dilemmas that arise from genetic testing.

Use of genetic information

The types of samples used in newborn medical screening are newborn blood samples. By definition, these blood samples contain a newborn's

DNA. The DNA collected is imprinted on filter paper and stored after the tests are complete. It is thus possible for the clinical agency collecting the sample and the laboratory performing the analysis to have access to an infant's DNA. In any other genetic testing site, the collection of a sample for DNA analysis is preceded by an in-depth counseling session. No blood sample is analyzed until the patient or patient's guardian provides evidence of informed consent for genetic testing.

Genetic testing in children is regarded as a special case. It is generally recommended that routine genetic testing of children be delayed until after the age of majority unless there are pressing reasons to test a minor child. Certainly the prevention of irreversible damage by some of the metabolic syndromes screened for in the Newborn Screening (NBS) panel would meet this criterion. But having a DNA sample readily available may tempt those performing the analysis to use that sample for other purposes. It seems logical that parents, who often are not informed of the routine newborn screening being performed on their infant, be asked to give consent for the use of their infant's samples for other purposes. Crouch and colleagues [5] note that DNA samples are the best source of newborn identification, and demonstrate that either umbilical cord blood or infant heel stick specimens are equally effective in providing DNA. They recommend that parents be given a card with their infant's DNA to be stored in a safe place for future use. Certainly it seems more appropriate that parents be the guardians of their infant's DNA than either hospitals or laboratories.

Ethics of performing a test when no treatment exists

With expanding technology, it is possible to test for hundreds of genetic conditions using the MS/MS assay. When there is neither a means of prevention nor an effective treatment of diagnosed conditions, the ethics of performing tests becomes a serious issue. Is it appropriate to have a one-size-fits-all model of newborn screening? It is important to have policy-level discussions regarding who gets to select and decide on the conditions that are screened. For example, consider the case of cystic fibrosis. The sensitivity and specificity of various panels of mutations depend on many variables, including ethnicity. Although the sensitivity and specificity in the Ashkenazi Jewish population is very high, the test is considerably

less reliable in Asian and African populations. The use of these tests and their interpretation can therefore have lifelong ramifications not only on quality of life but also on potential use of the information to deny health insurance or employment.

Inclusion of a family history tool in neonatal assessment and its significance

Another change in practice that has been encouraged by the Human Genome Project and supported by the former US Surgeon General Dr. Richard Carmona is to conduct a family history on all patients and families. The federal endorsement has been noted as taking a family history around a holiday time, such as Thanksgiving, so that it is a part of family traditions. From a health standpoint, many hidden genetic problems would be discovered by taking a three-generation family history. These forms are downloadable from http://www.hhs.gov/familyhistory/; for maternal–child nurses this tool should be part of the neonatal assessment to learn what might present in a newborn or infant's life. If this tool, which is straightforward and easy to use, were to be incorporated into health assessments and histories, the spirit of the original newborn screening to detect problems early, prevent complications when possible, and improve the quality of life would be upheld. But many times this tool is not used because of a concern about lack of time. That is why that the push should be for families to conduct their own histories and bring them to the health care provider. That would be the ideal, but we have to encourage and teach the public and ourselves to do that. So what is the bottom line for newborn genetic testing? Do families also need to realize that there are still risks to indiscriminate use of genetic information?

Genetic information nondiscrimination action legislation

As this article was being written lawmakers were considering the Genetic Information Non-discrimination Action of 2007 (GINA), H.R. 493/S. 358. The purpose of this bill is to ensure that every American can undergo genetic testing without fear of how that information will be used. The bill expressly protects the public from discrimination in employment or health insurance issues because of the existence of a genetic condition. This legislation was introduced in January 2007 and still has not passed. Although this bill is still pending it is in the public's interest to know that this is one of the risks for discrimination when genetic testing is done. This is another instance that may result in testing not being done that could improve a prognosis or quality of life. Conversely, it is another reason to be careful and clear about how, when, and where genetic testing, even on newborns, is done. Newborn testing is often so accepted as the standard of care that the same considerations by health professionals or even some families are not given to this form of genetic testing. So again, the question becomes "Just because we can, should we?"

Clinical implications

Oftentimes nurses in clinical practice are woefully underprepared to provide genetic education to parents and families. Currently there is an initiative to implement the *Essential Nursing Competencies and Curricula Guidelines for Genetics and Genomics* [6] into all levels of nursing education and clinical practice. This work is an extension of the National Coalition for Health Professional Education in Genetics (http://www.nchpeg.org/) that created competencies for all health professionals who touch a patient. These guidelines have been endorsed by more than 40 professional nursing associations along with several schools of nursing and not-for-profit agencies, such as the March of Dimes. Nurses at all levels of educational preparation, all specialties, and all clinical settings would be well-served to review these guidelines and use the resources provided to prepare themselves to provide safe and effective nursing care. It is clear that with the emphasis on genetic testing, the information that is readily available to the public coupled with the almost daily breakthroughs in genetic linkages with disease and genomic factors, including family history and environmental exposures that raise the risk for a genetic disease occurring, aggressive testing will become a standard of care. In many ways it already is in most states. If the test is not offered to the family or not run, we most likely suffer the liability of falling short of the acceptable standard of care. As health professionals, we need to be aware of the state of genetic testing and of what our role is in protecting the newborn and family from potential harm.

Genetic testing is more than screening. Screening clearly implies assessment and recognition of a problem, and generally is not involved in definitive diagnostic testing or treatment plans. Testing is broader. According to the National Human Genome Research Institute (http://www.nlm.nih.gov/medlineplus/genetictesting.html) the public wants testing to determine a disease condition based on a gene alteration or a risk for the development of a problem at some point in their lives, ideally while still in the presymptomatic stage. Now as more information is known about genomics interaction between genes and the environment or lifestyle choices and the development of diseases more people are requesting genetic testing. Other families are using the testing for identifying embryos that might have a genetic condition through a process called preimplantation genetic diagnosis and in preconception planning to determine if they are carriers for specific genetic diseases that might put their potential offspring at risk. Again the tricky part is to make sure the tests are run by a reliable laboratory and that there is a health professional genetic counselor or one knowledgeable in genetics to interpret the results accurately. There are also concerns about genetic testing kits that are available. Some are not reliable. This concern has grown to the point of having groups such as Quackwatch disseminate information on dubious gene testing (http://www.quackwatch.org/01Quack eryRelatedTopics/Tests?genomics.html). The genetic breakthroughs in testing have caused the Centers for Disease Control and Prevention to fund a project called "Evaluation of genomic applications in practice and Prevention (EGAPP): implementation and evaluation of a model approach" to establish and evaluate a process that is evidence-based to assess genetic testing (http://www.cdc.gov/genomics/gTesting.htm). This initiative is under the auspices of the National Office of Public Health Genomics. This office offers information on genetic testing and implications for rare diseases and single-gene problems. It also disseminates information about the ethical, social, and legal implications of such testing. Most of the EGAPP work to date has been in the adult population, with emphasis on cancer, but its principles can and should be applied to newborns and infants also. Another related concern is the cost. Most genetic tests run from several hundred to several thousand dollars. These tests may not be covered by health insurance. So have these tests become available (beyond the state-mandated tests) to only those families who can pay? Is this another example of an ethical dilemma caused by the regulation of our health care in the United States? The answer would seem to be yes. Newborn screening and genetic testing are commonplace and there are obvious advantages to some level of screening and testing if the prognosis or quality of life can be improved, but there is still a lot to learn about these new technologies and the ethical issues that surround their use. Health professionals must keep abreast of the changes and help consumers to make informed choices.

Summary

Newborn medical screening has evolved into genetic testing with an emphasis on health promotion and disease prevention. This development includes taking a family history to identify risk factors that can be addressed by advocating for healthier lifestyles or for more careful follow-up care than the infant and eventual adult without such risk would need. The ability to test and screen in a fairly noninvasive, cost-effective manner is possible, but if there is not a cure or the course of the disease cannot be altered should we do it? Should we put a family at risk for loss of health insurance or the individual for eventual loss of a job potential because of an identified risky condition? What should be done about tests that are inadvertently run because of misinformation, lack of regulation, or ignorance? These are just a few of the ethical and potentially legal questions raised by genetic testing. We must have a solid knowledge of the most current information regarding genetic testing of newborns and recognize the field is ever changing.

References

[1] Meier JH. Screening, assessment and intervention for young children at developmental risk. In: Friedlander BZ, Sterritt GM, Kirk GE, editors. Exceptional infant: assessment and intervention, vol. 3. New York: Brunner/Mazel; 1975. p. 605–50.

[2] Wald NJ, editor. Antenatal and neonatal screening. New York: Oxford University Press; 1984.

[3] Apgar V. A proposal for a new method of evaluation of the newborn infant. Curr Res Anesth Analg 1953; 32:260–7.

[4] Apgar V, Holaday DA, James LS, et al. Evaluation of the newborn infant—second report. J Am Med Assoc 1958;168:1985–8.

[5] Crouch SJ, Rowell KR, Beiser S. Umbilical cord blood for newborn DNA identification. J Obstet Gynecol Neonatal Nurs 2007;36:308–12.

[6] Consensus Panel on Genetic/Genomic Nursing Competencies. Essential nursing competencies and curricula guidelines for genetics and genomics. Silver Spring (MD): American Nurses Association; 2006.

[7] Littman G, Parmalee AH. Medical correlates of infant development. Pediatrics 1978;61:470–4.

[8] Frankenburg WK, Dodds JB. The Denver Developmental Screening Test. J Pediatr 1967;71:181–91.

[9] Frankenburg WK, Dodds JB, Archer P, et al. The Denver II: a major revision and restandardization of the Denver Developmental Screening Test. Pediatrics 1992;89:91–7.

[10] Noller K, Ingrisano D. Cross-sectional study of gross and fine motor development. Phys Ther 1984;64:308–16.

[11] The Associated Press. Nearly 90 percent of babies tested for genetic disorders. The Oklahoman July 2007. p. 22A. Available at: http://abcnews.go.com/Health/wireStory?id=3365185.

[12] National Human Genome Research Institute, Washington. About the human genome project. Updated August 2004. Available at: http://www.genome.gov/10001772. Accessed May 2, 2004.

[13] Kenner C, Moran M. Newborn screening and genetic testing. J Midwifery Womens Health 2005; 50(3):219–26.

[14] Kenner C, Gallo AM, Bryant KD. Promoting children's health through understanding of genetics and genomics. J Nurs Scholarsh 2005;37(4): 308–14.

[15] Little CM, Lewis JA. Newborn screening. Newborn and Infant Nursing Reviews 2008;8(1):3–9.

[16] American College of Medical Genetics. Newborn screening: toward a uniform screening panel and system. Available at: http://mchb.hrsa.gov/screening/summary.htm; 2005. Accessed June 18, 2007.

CRITICAL CARE
NURSING CLINICS
OF NORTH AMERICA

Crit Care Nurs Clin N Am 20 (2008) 239–243

Index

Note: Page numbers of article titles are in **boldface** type.